Life Hacks

Life Hacks

The King of Random's Tips and Tricks to Make Everyday Tasks Fun and Easy

- -

Grant Thompson
and
Instructables.com

Introduction by Wade Wilgus

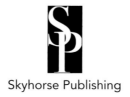

Skyhorse Publishing

Skyhorse Publishing books may be purchased in bulk at special discounts for sales promotion, corporate gifts, fund-raising, or educational purposes. Special editions can also be created to specifications. For details, contact the Special Sales Department, Skyhorse Publishing, 307 West 36th Street, 11th Floor, New York, NY 10018 or info@ skyhorsepublishing.com.

Skyhorse® and Skyhorse Publishing® are registered trademarks of Skyhorse Publishing, Inc.®, a Delaware corporation.

www.skyhorsepublishing.com

10 9 8 7 6 5 4 3 2 1

Library of Congress Cataloging-in-Publication Data is available on file.

Cover design by Owen Corrigan

Cover photos by Grant Thompson

Print ISBN: 978-1-62914-588-4

Ebook ISBN: 978-1-63220-025-9

Printed in China

Table of Contents

table of contents

Introduction

Grant Thompson, the King of Random, knows what his subjects want to see. He earned his crown with seemingly random projects and videos that led to an audience of millions across Youtube, Instructables, Facebook, and anywhere else that fascinating and fun content can be shared. A mad scientist with an eye toward making the world an amusing, interesting, and participatory experience, there's nothing random about the King.

Grant's projects work so well because they expose unfamiliar but awesome facets of everyday things that most people just consume or ignore. His projects are simple, clear, and easy to try at home. Some are frivolous, but most are clever responses to common problems. You may not need to make soap from drain cleaner and bacon or rig a stick welder from microwave components. But the King of Random will show you how anyway.

In this book, you'll find novel ways to enjoy summer, prepare and consume food, celebrate the holidays, save money, play with ice, save energy, work with metal, and discover other tweaks and adjustments that make life easier or more fun.

And who doesn't want their life to be easier and more fun?

What is Instructables?

Instructables.com is a bona fide Internet sensation, a web-based community of motivated do-it-yourselfers who contribute invaluable how-to guides to the site on a wide range of topics, from gardening and home repair to recipes to gadgets that defy categorization. The site hosts more than 100,000 projects. More than fifteen million people visit the site each month, leaving comments and suggestions on the ever-growing list of do-it-yourself projects.

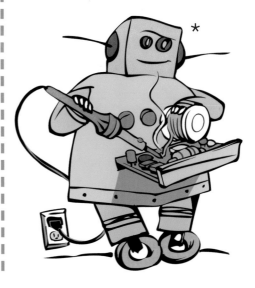

*

* Special thanks to Instructables Interactive Designer Gary Lu for the Instructables Robot illustrations!

Section 1
Summer Hacks

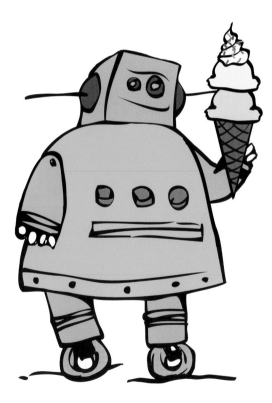

Icy Drinks Every Time

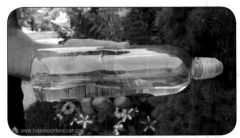

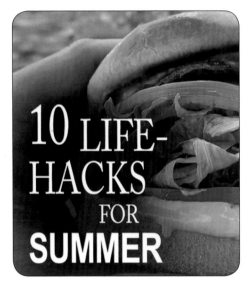

10 LIFE-HACKS FOR SUMMER

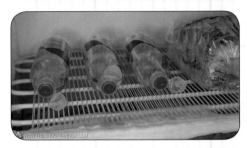

Here are ten amazing tips and tricks you can use to impress your friends and make your summer a little easier.

I wrote this in hopes that all of you would enjoy this compilation of ten "life hacks" that has helped and inspired me.

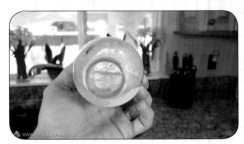

I found many of them on sites such as LifeHacker.com, Pinterest.com, and Google.com. The mango and fruit fly projects were inspired by my wife from a trick she learned while visiting Argentina.

WARNING:

These projects and results are depictions of my own personal experiences. Your results may vary depending on your location and modifications to project ideas. There may be risks associated with some of these projects that require adult supervision.

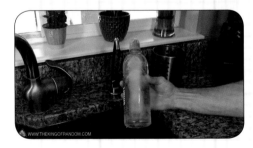

When you need a drink to cool down, hot water can taste disgusting. Try filling your water bottles a quarter of the way, so that when they're on their sides, the water settles just below the bottle neck. Now stick your bottles in the freezer and go on with your day. When the water is frozen it will make an ice block on the side of the bottle, but doesn't block the opening. Now when you need to cool off, just take a bottle from the freezer, fill it up with your favorite drink, and you've got an instant icy cold beverage ready to go.

Mango Hack

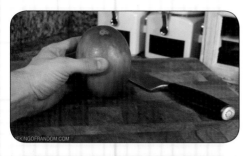

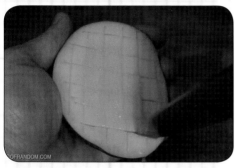

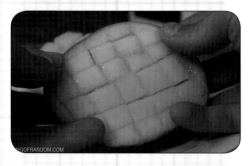

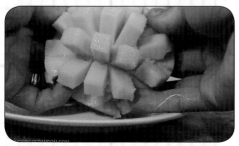

Grab yourself a mango and try this little trick. Carefully cut off the two sides of the fruit and hold one piece in your hand. You can gently cut a few lines vertically and a few more horizontally until the pattern resembles a checkerboard. Now take it with both hands and gently push from the back. You'll see bite-sized pieces pop right up and they're ready to eat. You can use a spoon to scrape them into a bowl or just eat them right off the peel. It's fast, easy, and they won't get stuck in your teeth.

Eat Your Hamburger Upside-Down

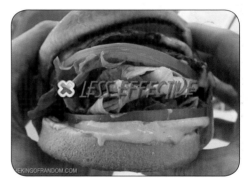

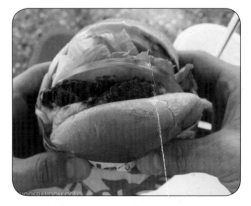

The next time you eat a giant hamburger, try turning your sandwich upside down. The tops are nearly twice as thick as the bottoms and a lot more durable, so be smart and eat your hamburgers upside-down.

3

Anti-Ant Hack

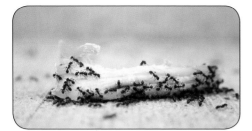

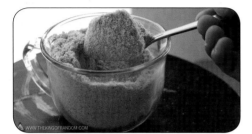

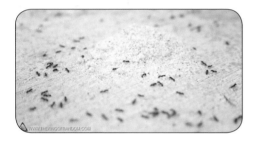

Covert Container

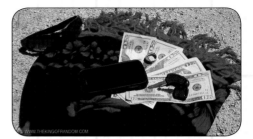

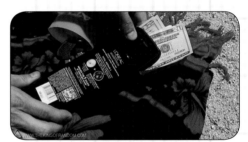

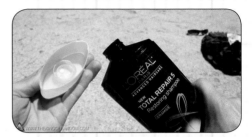

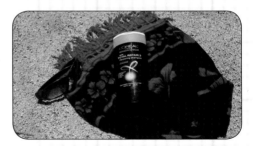

If you've got ants and you're looking for a natural form of pest control, try measuring out a cup of popcorn kernels. Put them in a blender on high speed for about thirty seconds and you'll end up with a batch of fresh homemade cornmeal. Just make a few piles around the ant trails, and within a few days, your ant problems will literally disappear.

When you're at the beach, reduce the chances of things getting stolen by making a covert container. Just take your old shampoo bottle and twist the top so that it pops right off. Clean it out and cut a hole in the top that's just big enough to stash your valuable items inside. Now you can snap the top back on and your items are perfectly concealed. Anyone who sees this will just think it's a shampoo bottle, and chances are, nobody wants to steal your shampoo.

Soda Cans and Straws

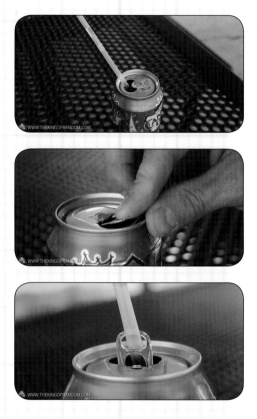

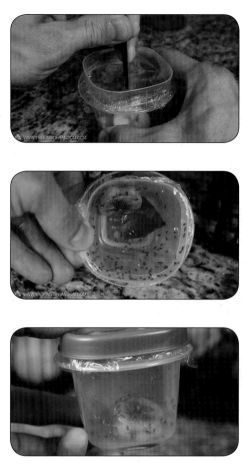

Have you ever noticed that when you put a straw in a can of soda, it doesn't want to stay? Try bending the tab of the can over the hole and sliding your straw down through the tab. No more floating straws, because now it's held in place.

Fruit Fly Hack

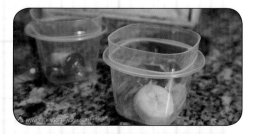

It's the season for fruit flies, so before they take over your kitchen, slice a few pieces of banana and mix them with some of your leftover mango peels. Find a couple of small containers and add the fruit. Now just stretch a piece of plastic wrap over the top and use something like the tip of a chopstick to poke a small hole in the center that's just bigger than the fly. Now you can set it and forget about it. Within a few minutes, the flies will be checking things out, and once one goes in, you can be sure his friends will follow. Within a couple of days, they'll all be having a rocking fruit party. And now you can simply take the lid of the container and press it on, sealing them inside. Now you are the lord of the flies.

Dripping Popsicle Fix

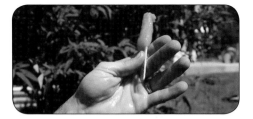

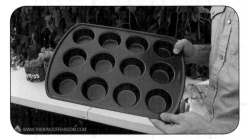

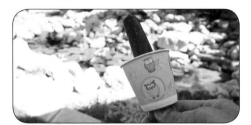

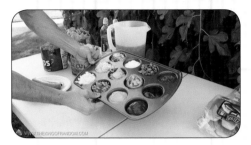

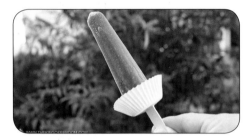

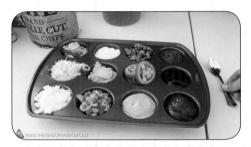

Summer means popsicles, and popsicles mean your kids are going to get sticky fingers. Grab a small paper cup, and carefully poke a hole in the bottom, about the size of a popsicle stick. Now when you push a popsicle inside, you've got an instant drip catcher and no more sticky fingers. By the way, this works great with cupcake liners as well!

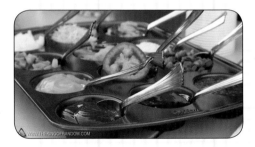

Quick and Clean Condiments

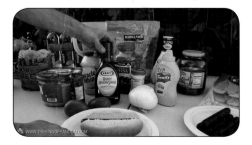

You've probably been to a barbecue where the condiments take up half the table, and the lineups for using them take forever. Solve the problem with a muffin pan. This way, your condiments are easy to access and your lines will move along quickly. You'll also dramatically increase your table space and cut down on the things to clean up afterward.

Instant Snack Bowl

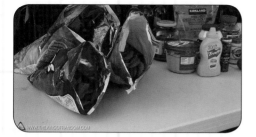

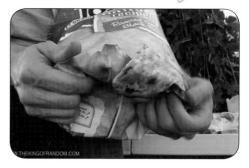

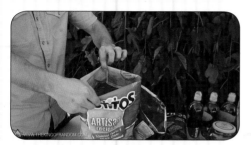

The next time you're at a party and someone has bags of chips lying around, impress your friends by making them into custom snack bowls. You can fold the top edge inside the bag first, then begin rolling the bottom corners, up into the base of the bag, pushing the chips up as you go. You'll end up with a custom snack bowl with chips overflowing.

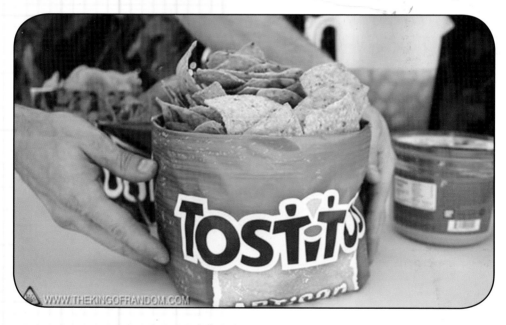

How to Make a PVC Water/Air/ Vacuum Pump!

In this project, you'll learn how to make a customizable PVC hand pump that will create vacuum suction, pump water, or compress air. A pre-requisite to making the pump will be two homemade check valves.

WARNING:

Power tools, like a table saw, pose risks of serious injury. Adequate training and experience are required before operating. The results and claims of this pump are based solely on my personal experiences. Individual results may vary. The pump is a simple design and not made to be used in any heavy-duty operations or relatively high pressures. Use of this content is at your own risk.

Step 1: What You'll Need

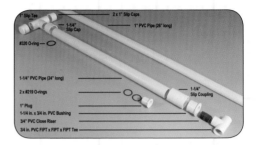

Whether you're using vacuum power, moving water, or compressing air, chances are you're using some type of a pump.

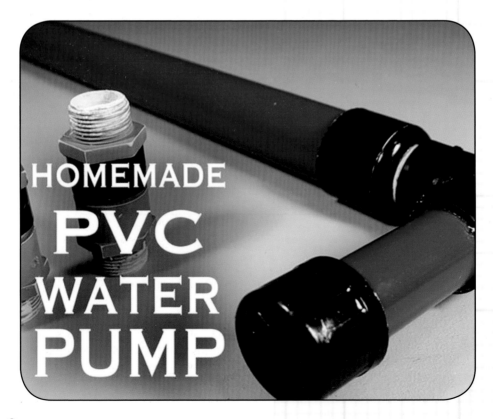

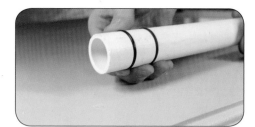

I thought it might be good to build a simple pump, mainly for learning purposes, and I wanted to do it with low-cost materials.

I've wanted to build a PVC water pump for awhile, but the check valves were around ten dollars each. That seemed a little steep for a PVC build, so I made my own.

I was inspired on the pump piston and chamber by a picture I saw on a Google image search by someone who used the 1¼" and 1" sizes of tubes, and he mentioned he cut the grooves for the O ring on a table saw. That was a new idea to me and gave me the inspiration to put this together.

The materials I used are outlined in detail in the picture.

Step 2: Making the Piston

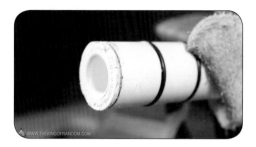

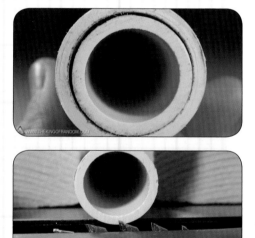

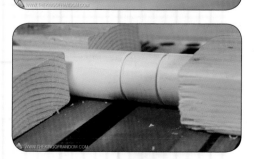

You can see here that the 1" pipe fits closely inside of the 1¼" PVC pipe. There is just a little gap, but we actually need this to be air-tight to make a proper piston. The best way that I know to make an air-tight seal is by using some rubber O ring.

To cut grooves for the rings, I used a table saw and adjusted the blade by holding the pipe flat on the table top and lowering the blade until I could see that it would only cut about halfway through the plastic. The goal is to make a nice groove for the O ring, but not to compromise the structural integrity of the PVC pipe too much.

I cut two grooves for redundancy. One at 1" and another at the 2" mark.

I used some wooden braces to keep the pipe steady and made the cuts by using one hand to hold the pipe on the blade and the other hand to rotate the pipe slowly. (Of course, safety and caution are top priorities when working around power tools and open cutting blades.) The O ring fit perfectly into place.

This end of the pipe also needs to be capped off to seal it air-tight.

You can't really tell in the picture, but I've glued on an end plug that is solid. In the diagram, I said it was a 1" plug, but in reality it was a ¾" plug that I sanded down to fit inside the end of this 1" pipe.

Now this end of the tube is completely sealed.

Step 3: Finishing the Piston and Chamber

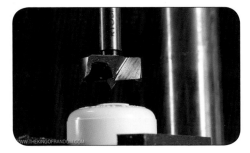

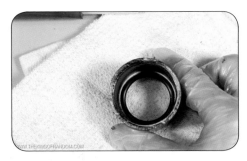

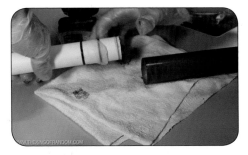

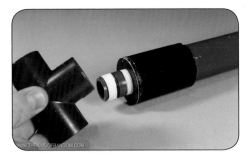

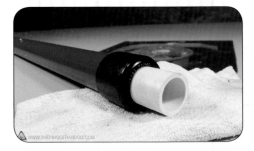

To finish the piston, we need to do a little work on the exterior tube.

I got a 1¼" slip cap and used a 1⅜" Forstner bit to drill a hole in the center.

An O ring was added into the inside of the cap around the hole, and put to the side for a minute. To insert the piston, the O ring need some lubrication or the friction on the inside walls of the pipe will damage them. I used Vaseline, but some people have suggested Vaseline will eat the O ring over time, and that some type of silicon grease would be better.

To the bottom of the 1¼" pipe I cemented on the coupling, ¾" reducer bushing, short riser, and threaded tee. With the two O ring lubricated, the piston should push air-tight into the larger pipe.

The modified slip cap can be cemented on top now, and when the piston is bottomed out, there should just be a couple of inches of pipe poking out the top.

Step 4: Painting and Cementing

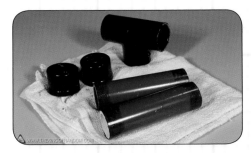

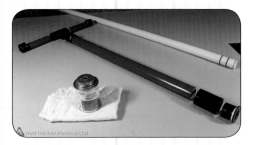

I chose to paint the fittings black and the pipe blue, just for contrast.

The handle is made from two pieces of 4½" x 1" PVC pipe cut from the scraps off of the piston.

Everything is cemented together as shown in the picture, and when the handle is complete, it cements onto those couple of inches of piston pipe sticking out of the hydraulic piston chamber.

This completes the piston, and adding two check valves to the threaded Tee at the bottom will complete the pump!

NOTE:

Make sure your check valves are pointing the right way.

Step 5: Testing the Pump

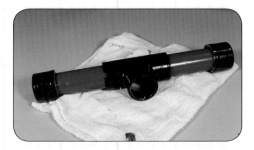

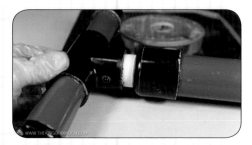

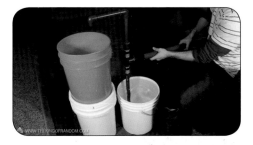

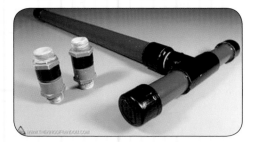

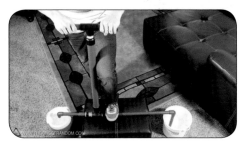

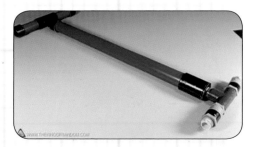

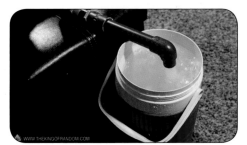

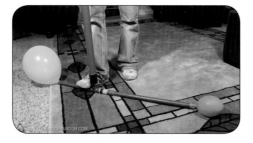

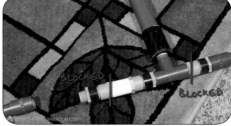

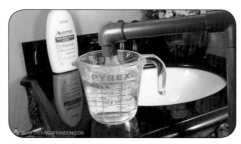

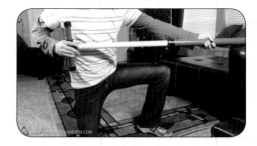

Since the check valves are threaded, they can be moved around, changed out, or positioned in many creative ways.

Using additional PVC pipe and fittings opens up many different options. The imagination is the limitation.

You could try making this into a pump to move water vertically, or leverage it with your feet for more of a bilge pump type approach. This pump seemed to move just over two cups of water per cycle.

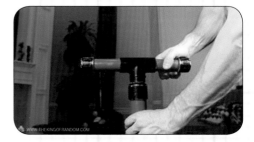

With the vertical pump approach, I could pump around three gallons per minute. With the horizontal approach, I could move over five gallons per minute because I could put my weight into it and move it faster.

Step 6: Additional Features

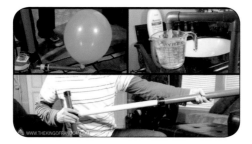

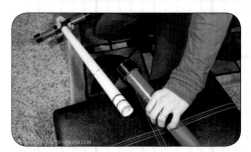

The pump was made for pumping water, but it proves extremely effective for compressing air as well as creating a vacuum. The pump has an intake side, and an outflow side. If you hook up to the intake, you create a vacuum.

I blew up a balloon and attached it to the intake side, and on every stroke it got smaller and smaller until it was actually sucked inside the tube. I tried blocking the valves from both directions, and when I pulled back on the piston, I was met with a strong vacuum in the chamber, which pulled the piston back inside with considerable force when I let go.

Because the piston isn't physically attached to anything, the handle can rotate a full 360 degrees.

If you need to clean the piston, or add some more lubrication, you can pull the whole handle out like an oversized plunger. It goes back in the same way it came out.

I'm planning to use this piston design in future projects that require pneumatic and hydraulic pistons.

In my testing, the valves work great with air and water. I didn't have any gauges to test the strength of the vacuum so can't say how strong the vacuum would be, but it certainly does create one.

Step 7: Final Thoughts

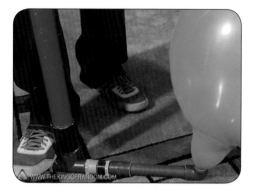

While there are some special tools used to create this pump (table saw and Forstner drill bit), I believe that with a little creativity, the pump could be made just as effectively without them, making this a simple and easy-to-duplicate design.

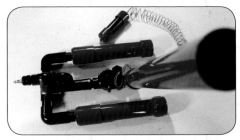

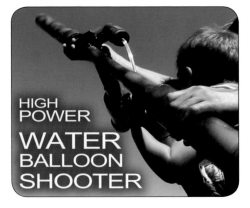

HIGH POWER WATER BALLOON SHOOTER

Bring out the big guns!

Have you ever seen a water balloon shotgun? Here's how to make a high-power water balloon shooter that will fire seventeen balloons at once!

WARNING:

Adult supervision and adequate training is recommended. Misuse or careless use of equipment or projects may result in serious injury, property damage, and/or death. Use of content is at your own risk.

Rocket Rifle and Candy Cannon

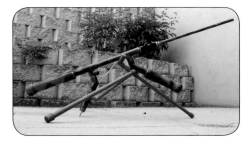

This project is a done with a simple modification to some of my previous projects. This will also work with the "Candy Cannon" (page 34), and no modification is necessary.

Step 1: Modify the Rocket Rifle with the Cannon Adaptor

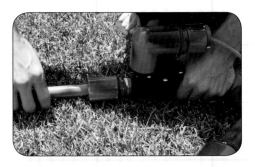

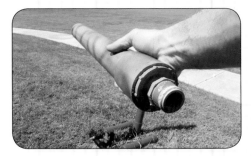

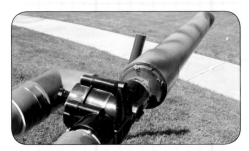

To modify the Rocket Rifle into a Water Balloon Shotgun, all you'll need to do is unscrew the barrel and replace it with the Cannon Adaptor.

The Cannon Adaptor is simply a 2' length of 2" PVC pipe, a 2" coupling, and some reducer bushings to bring the threads down to 1". Lastly, a 1" close (short) PVC riser so it will screw into the sprinkler valve on the rifle. I added some camouflage paint to match the gun.

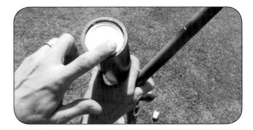

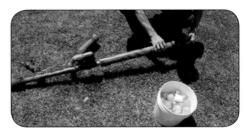

Step 2: Shooting Water Balloons

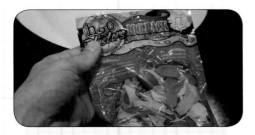

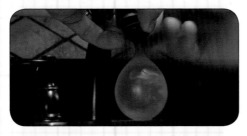

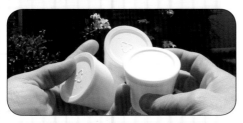

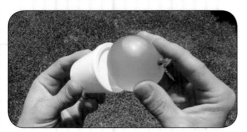

When shooting water balloons, one challenge you need to be aware of is the possibility that the pressure from the gun bursts the balloon before it even gets out of the barrel.

There are four steps you can take to get a successful launch.

1. Wadding:

You need something that will cushion the pressure on the balloon as it's launched. I made some wads with plastic cups. They are firm but cushion the balloon enough during the acceleration to keep it intact. You could also use cloth or even as something as simple as a moistened rolled up sock.

You can use the barrel from your rocket rifle as a ram-rod to push the wad to the bottom of the barrel. It should be as close to an air-tight fit as you can get.

2. Lubrication:

If the barrel is dry, the balloon will pop when it's fired. This is because of the friction during payload acceleration.

I found that using a bit of vegetable oil to coat the sides of the barrel eliminated this problem. It also helps lubricate the diaphragm in the sprinkler valve to prevent it from locking up.

Water works as lubrication as well, but over time, the minerals from the water will dry inside the valve and may make it lock up at higher pressures to the point where the 9V battery isn't strong enough to open it.

3. Size of balloon:

The smaller the balloon, the stronger it will be. I had great results with balloons that had a slightly smaller diameter than the barrel. If they are wider than the barrel, you can still make them fit, but there will be more friction as they exit, and a greater chance of failure.

4. Using the right pressure:

I found that 65–70 PSI works great for a single water balloon. At this pressure, you can expect a balloon to fly around 300 feet!

You can fit multiple balloons in the barrel and will need to adjust the pressure up slightly with each one you add. I tested all the way up to seventeen balloons at 90 PSI with great results!

Step 3: Seventeen Water Balloons at Once!

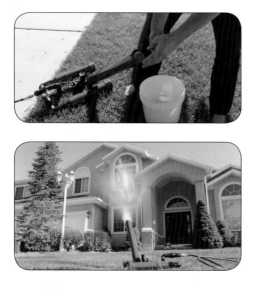

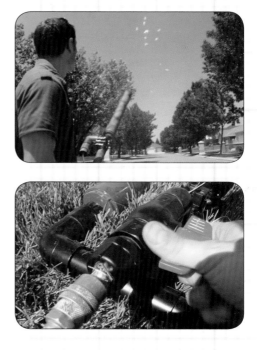

A 2' barrel will hold around seventeen water balloons. This increases the weight of the payload significantly, so a pressure of around 90+ PSI is recommended for long-distance shots. Otherwise, they will just plop out of the end. Funny, but not very effective.

There is quite a bit of kick as the balloons are fired out, so using the Candy Cannon as a Water Balloon Mortar is the easiest option, and the barrel can be tilted for trajectory. However, using the Rocket Rifle to shoot multiple balloons has a great and powerful feeling to it that you can't get with the Candy Cannon.

For portability, the manual ball valve near the fill port can be closed, maintaining the pressure charge in your water weapon. It will probably only be good for one shot, but will give you the option to disconnect from the air hose and go anywhere. The pressure charge should hold indefinitely.

Homemade Sparklers for the Fourth of July! Improvised Handheld Fireworks

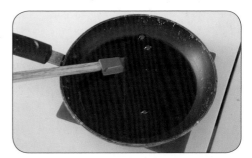

(DIY PYRO)

HOME-BREW SPARKLERS

In this project, we're making handheld sparklers for the Fourth of July. When it's time to celebrate with fireworks, you could just buy them. Or you could improvise and make your own.

WARNING:

There is a very real risk to health and safety. This project should not be attempted without adult supervision and adequate training. Pyrotechnics are not toys and should be handled with extreme caution and respect. High temperatures on the stove or oven may cause auto-ignition of the pyrotechnic composition, which may lead to serious injury, death, and/or permanent damage to equipment and property. Ignition of an incendiary or explosive material may not be legal in your area, and resulting damage may not be covered by your insurance. Check city laws and ordinances before attempting.

Step 1: Sparkle Stick Recipe

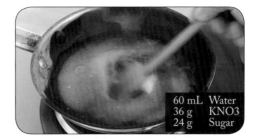

60 mL	Water
36 g	KNO3
24 g	Sugar

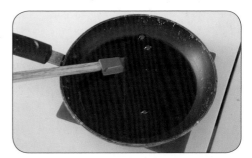

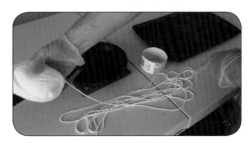

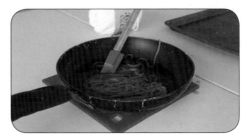

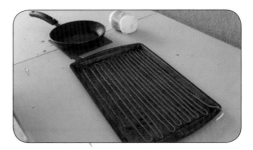

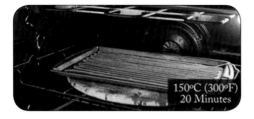

150°C (300°F)
20 Minutes

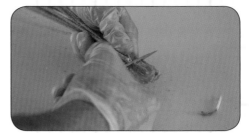

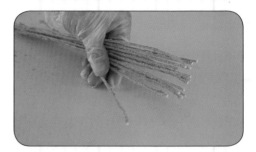

This sparkler, or sparkle stick, works best at night or in low-light conditions. During the day, you see more smoke than you do sparks, but both effects are pretty fun.

This is the recipe for making a "sparkle stick":

• 60 mL water (heated on medium heat)

• 36 grams KNO3 (potassium nitrate), which I obtained in the form of stump remover

• 24 grams white sugar

• 1–20 drops of food coloring (color to suit your preference)

NOTE:

White/gray smoke is the only color emitted, even if you use different colored dyes. Colored smoke cannot be made with KNO3.

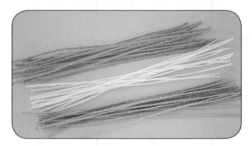

Shake the sugar and KNO3 together to get an intimate mixture, then pour into the water and stir until dissolved.

Soak about 12 feet of 100 percent cotton yarn in the solution, then space evenly on a cookie tray.

Bake in an oven at 150°C (300°F) for about twenty minutes, making sure to lift the yarn at ten minutes to make sure it doesn't stick to the pan.

Let cool for five to ten minutes.

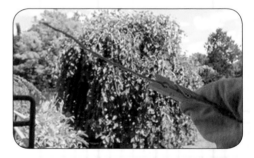

Step 2: Cut to Desired Sizes

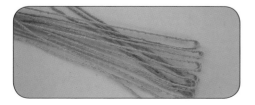

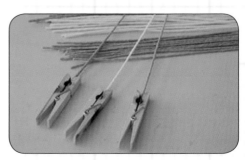

When your sparkle cords are cooled down, you can easily cut them to any desired size with a pair of scissors and place in clothespin. I made a couple of different batches in different colors for the holiday.

Step 3: Lighting Your Sparklers

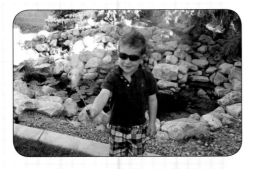

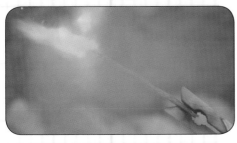

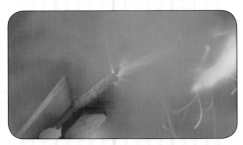

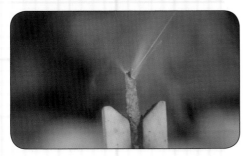

Now you can put on gloves and safety glasses, light your sparkler, and enjoy!

Gloves are recommended as bits of burning fuel will occasionally fly off and can burn the skin.

If the sparkler burns too fast, wait a few hours or days to try again. The composition is hygroscopic and will absorb moisture from the air, reducing the rate of burn until eventually it won't light at all.

If you want to revive an old batch that has absorbed too much moisture, re-bake in the oven for twenty minutes at 150°C (300°F).

These types of devices may not be legal to make or use in your area, so check local laws before attempting to duplicate this project, and as always, be safe and aware of your environment before igniting anything flammable!

Enjoy!

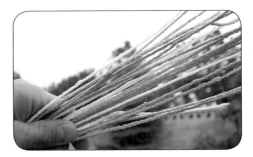

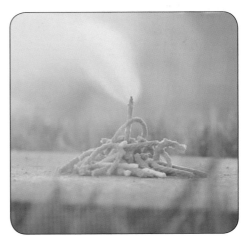

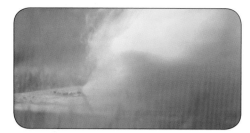

The best part is that you can make hundreds of these sparklers for only a few dollars, and the clippings can be burned together for a more dramatic display!

Well, now you know how to make some improvised handheld fireworks to celebrate your special occasion.

Section 2
Food Hacks

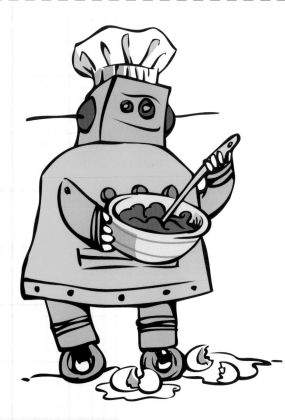

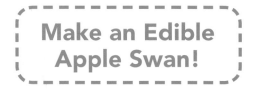
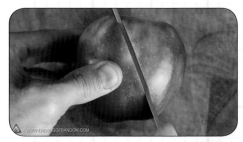

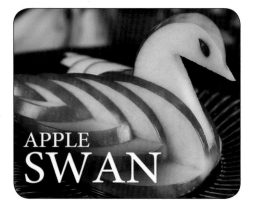

APPLE
SWAN

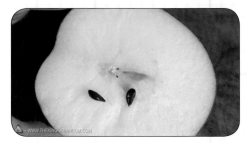

How to make a decorative, and completely edible, apple swan! I made a few modifications to the original idea, to get the effect you see here.

WARNING:

There may be risks associated with these projects that require adult supervision.

All you really need for this little trick is an apple and a knife. Two additional butter knives are helpful, but optional. Try cutting your apple at a slight diagonal so that it cuts right through the center of the apple core. This is important because it will give you access to the seeds inside, and we need two. You'll see why later on.

Step 1: Choose Your Apple

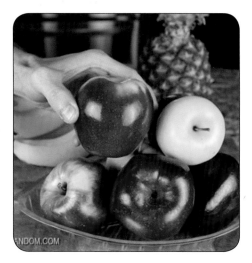

Step 2: Making Apple Wedges

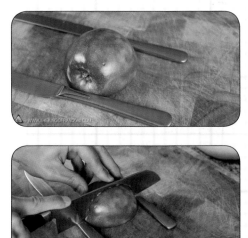

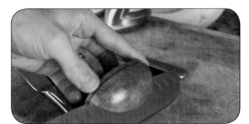

Step 3: Give it Wings!

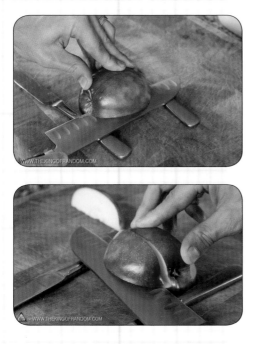

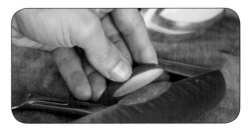

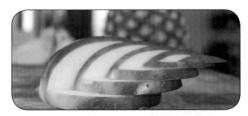

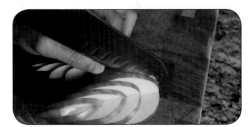

Take the half of the apple that still has the bottom attached and place it face down on a cutting board.

We're going to be making careful cuts into the apple, and I found it was very helpful to use two butter knives placed perpendicular to the top and bottom.

Now use your knife to carefully cut down into the apple from the top, and just to the right side of the apple core. You should be able to press down until the knife bottoms out on the other two butter knives, and then use the butter knives as makeshift spacers to line your knife up, and cut in from the side.

When the two cuts meet, you may feel a little "pop" as the wedge is released. If not, it means the cuts haven't fully met yet, so just gently wiggle the blade from both directions until the cuts align.

Repeat the process on the other side of the apple so that you're left with two apple wedges similar to those seen in the pictures.

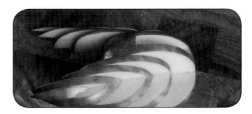

The goal is to cut each of these new wedges into three smaller wedges, then layer them together to give the effect of feathers and wings.

The process is very similar to how you cut them before, but this time, rather than slicing in from the side, try turning the wedge over to the left, and slicing down. This should give you more control and save you a few potential cuts to your fingers.

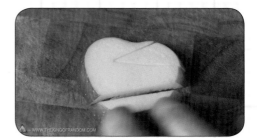

When both wedges have been cut, layer the pieces back together to form a teardrop shape, and replace them back into the apple "body." The effect should be two beautiful swan wings.

We still need to make a place for the head to sit, so make a couple of precision cuts near the front of the body and remove the pieces to leave a clean and fairly deep groove, as seen in the picture.

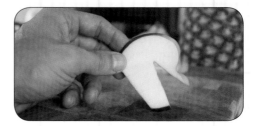

Step 4: Making the Head

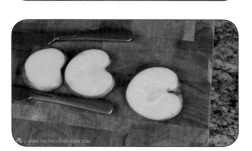

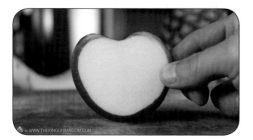

To form the head, we can use the other half of the apple and place it in-between our butterknife spacers as we did the other one, except this time we're not going to cut out any wedges.

Carefully cut sideways along the butter knives to create an apple slice about ¼" thick. If you repeat this three or four times, you'll end up with different cross sections that sport a variety of shapes and sizes.

Pick a piece that looks like a heart that's been flattened at the top. I've found these shapes work the best.

All we need to form the head are three strategic cuts into the apple slice. I made one cut at the top at about a 45-degree angle, then a second cut horizontal and to the right. The last cut near the bottom was sloped at about 30 degrees down and to the left. You should be able to see that the top cut was started just on the other side of the apple center, and this is done on purpose to give the sloped face, and the effect of a swan's beak.

Holding the piece up now should leave you with something similar to the picture.

24

Step 5: Putting It All Together

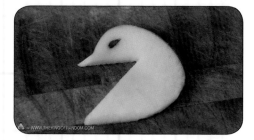

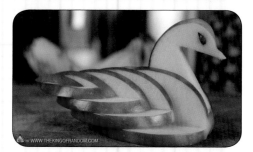

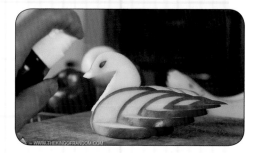

To finish up, just take your apple seeds and place them where you'd like the eyes to go, then press them into place with the side of one of the butter knives.

When both eyes are in place, simply drop the neck down into place, and your apple swan is finished!

I tried spritzing mine with a little lemon juice to help prevent it from turning brown, then we set it out for entertaining guests we have over for dinner that evening

Step 6: Variations

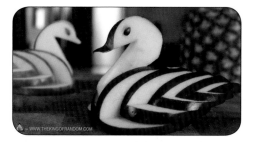

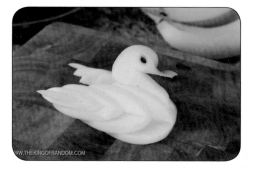

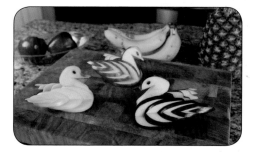

If you try this with different apples, you get different looking birds. No two birds will look exactly the same. In fact, I think some of mine look more like ducks.

Healthier Living by Making Butter (Shaking Cream into Butter)

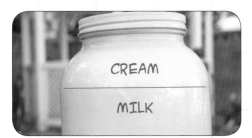

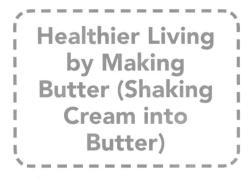

Healthy living just got a little butter. Caution: Shaking cream into butter makes people laugh at you.

NOTE:

This method takes five to ten minutes, but Dan Rojas with GreenPowerScience found a way to make the butter in under a minute by using a water bottle.

WARNING:

Use safe practices when handling food to avoid contamination, and only use milk or cream from trusted and approved sources. Shaking cream into butter may result in an amazing workout.

Step 1: Get Some Heavy Cream or Whipping Cream

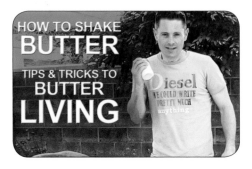

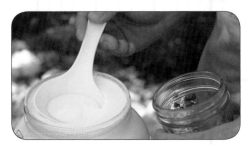

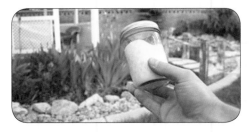

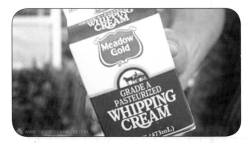

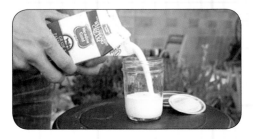

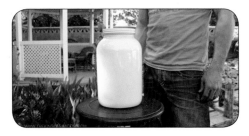

For this project, I decided to try making butter with milk I got straight from the cow.

My wife knows a lady with a cow, so one night we stopped by and picked up a gallon. After letting it sit in the refrigerator overnight, we could see a faint line showing where the cream had risen to the top with the milk underneath.

The trick is to skim the cream off the top and capture it into a container. I used a wide-mouth mason jar.

NOTE:

If you don't have access to a cow, a heavy cream or whipping cream will work just as well.

Step 2: Butter Churning—1

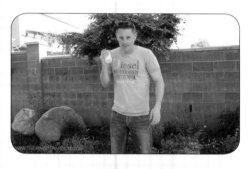

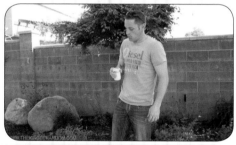

All you have to do to make cream into butter is shake it.

The method that worked well for me was to shake the jar up and down for two to three minutes as hard and as quickly as I could.

If you're using whipping cream, then after three minutes you shouldn't hear any more sloshing around in the jar. If you take the lid off to peek inside, you should find that it's turned to a light and fluffy whipped cream.

You could add a little sugar and stop here if you wanted. But if you want butter, you'll need to continue on.

Reminder: This method takes a little while because the sides of the jar are smooth.

Step 3: Butter Churning—2

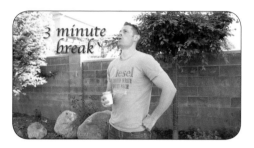

When your cream has turned to whipping cream, feel free to take a three-minute break.

This seems to help the whipping cream settle to the bottom a bit, making the next step a lot easier and quicker.

Step 4: Butter Churning—3

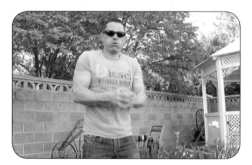

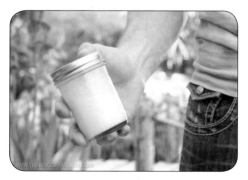

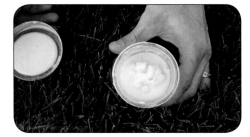

we got from the store. Can you see the difference? The homemade butters are at the top and right of the last picture.

Step 5: Traditional Buttermilk and Honey Butter

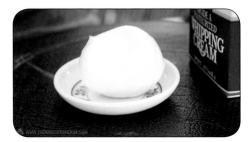

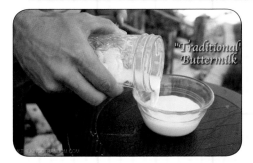

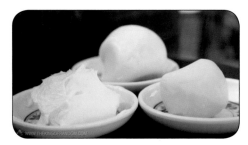

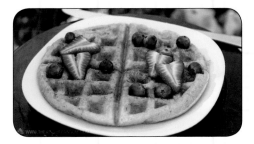

Shake as hard and as fast as you can! You are on the home-stretch to getting butter. The harder and faster you shake, the quicker the cream is going to break. When you begin to hear liquid sloshing around in the jar again, you're almost done. Just shake a little bit longer to make sure it's all complete.

This time when you look in the jar, you should see two distinct substances—a ball of something creamy and yellow and some liquid. The creamy yellow ball is butter and is ready to eat! It should be good for a couple of days, but if you want it to last longer, rinse it in cold water until the water turns clear and mix in a pinch of salt. It can last around two weeks.

I compared this homemade butter with some of the highest quality butter

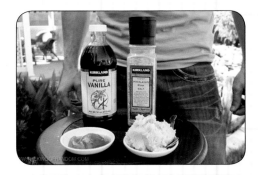

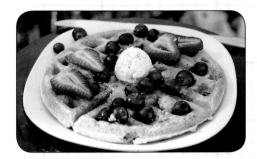

The excess liquid is "traditional buttermilk."

We tried using this to make whole wheat buttermilk waffles and they turned out great.

I used some raw organic honey and a few other ingredients, like vanilla and salt to make delicious honey butter. By the way, this tastes amazing on your fresh buttermilk waffles!

How to Make a Self-Freezing Coca-Cola (or Any Instant-Soda Slurpee)

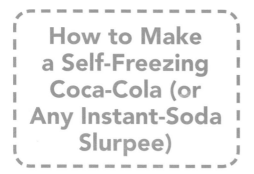

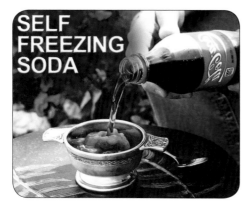

Make any bottle of soda freeze on command! This "super cool" trick works with cans of soda as well. I knew water could be turned to instant ice, but was amazed to see that soda could be super-cooled as well.

WARNING:

Leaving soda in the freezer too long can result in failure of the container and a big mess. Glass bottles are not recommended, as the ice expands when freezing and can shatter the glass explosively.

Self-Freezing Soda

The anomaly of "self-freezing soda" has been observed by many people, usually by accident.

Some people put a soda in the freezer to chill it but then forget about it. When they've remembered and gone to get it, it's liquid until they open it, leaving them puzzled. Some people

have noticed the effect by leaving the soda outside in cold temperatures.

There is a vending machine in Hong Kong that sells super-cooled Coke bottles, and the instructions to trigger nucleation is the same as in this video, however they recommend taking a sip when the cap is on. I believe this is to increase the chances of impurities being introduced into the liquid, making nucleation more likely.

From what I've seen, the results in this experiment form an even thicker slush than the vending machine in Hong Kong.

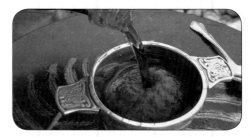

Super-cool Your Soda

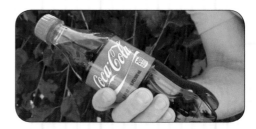

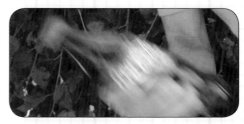

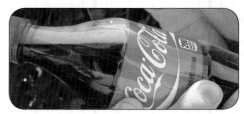

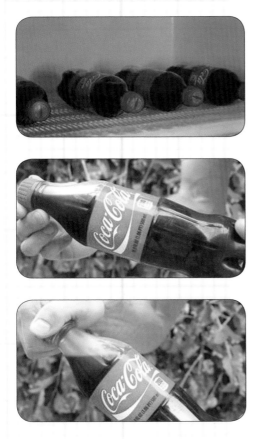

−24°C (−11°F) and takes three hours and fifteen minutes to super-chill four bottles.

Remember that the longer the freezer door is open, the more cold air will escape, and it will make your freeze times take much longer because your freezer has to cool down again. I've also noticed that the more frozen items you have in your freezer, the faster your soda will chill. In contrast, the fewer items in your freezer, the longer your soda will take to cool. Bottom line is that if you use a consistent environment for your experiments, you'll get consistent results!

The trick to getting the three-second slush is quickly releasing the pressure in the bottle and re-securing the cap, flipping the bottle upside-down and back upright again. This is because the forming ice crystals will be moved around the length of the bottle and trigger nucleation for the rest of the soda.

If you were to just take the cap off, ice will form, and it will slowly spread downward, but might take upwards of two minutes for the bottle to completely freeze.

Things to Try

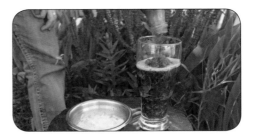

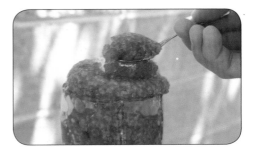

To get this effect, I shook up four bottles of 500 mL (16.9 oz) soda in a freezer set at −11°F (−24°C) for between three hours and fifteen minutes to four hours. The longer they are in, the more dramatic and solid the slushy freeze will be. However, any longer than three hours and fifteen minutes increases the chance of them freezing before you take them out. Shaking them up increases the pressure in the bottle, and actually lowers the freezing point a little.

Every freezer will be a little different temperature, and I've noticed the location of your bottles in the freezer makes a dramatic difference on freeze times. For best results, choose one consistent location in your freezer, and play around with freeze times to see what works best for you. In my freezer, the middle of the center rack settles at

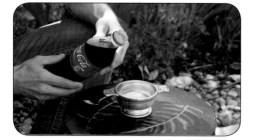

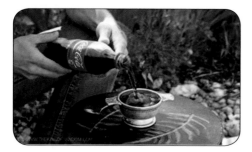

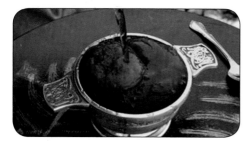

syrup would be more concentrated due to all the water that was taken out from it.

I found that if you opened the cap just enough to hear the bottle hissing and held it there until it stopped, you could remove the cap completely and the soda would stay a liquid.

I put a metal bowl in the freezer for about thirty minutes, and when it came out, it got frosty from the moisture in the air. If you pour your super-cooled soda into a frosty bowl, it's enough of a nucleation point to trip the ice crystallization, and you'll be able to pour yourself an "instant slushy."

Some people have asked what would happen if you were to drink a super-cooled soda. Simple answer is that it's cool and refreshing!

As the soda ices, latent heat is released in the crystallization and it actually warms up to just below freezing. That's similar to just having a drink with ice cubes floating in it, so go ahead and enjoy it!

More Things to Try

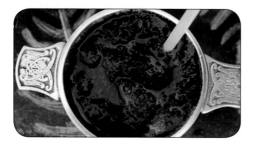

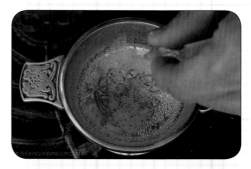

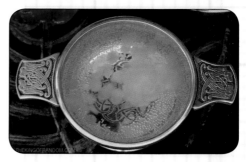

Once you've iced your soda, try pouring it into a glass to see how slushy it really is. It has a consistency similar to that of a Slurpee.

It's actually the water that is forming the ice crystals, and you'll notice the ice will begin to float to the top, trapping some of the soda syrup, and making delicious carbonated ice slush. If you were to remove the ice, the rest of the

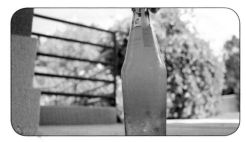

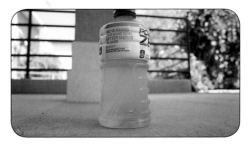

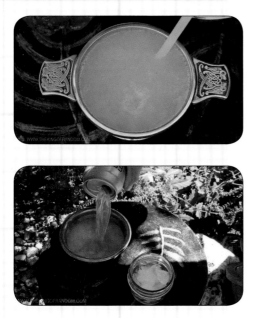

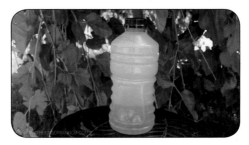

If you try pouring your super-cooled soda into a regular clean bowl or glass, it will just look like regular soda.

Now drop a flake of ice or ice cube into the liquid. As if by magic, the soda will crystallize until the whole bowl becomes slush. There's one tasty treat ready for serving!

This also works with cans of soda as well, but it is tougher. The freeze time is about the same, and the key to making it work is releasing the pressure from the can very, very slowly. This is much harder to do than opening a tab, but it is possible, and the soda has the same properties as the stuff from the bottles, obviously.

Other Experiments

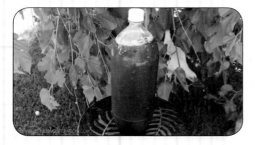

I also experimented with two-liter bottles and had great results freezing them between four and five hours. The whole bottle becomes slushy in an instant if you shake it upside down for a second.

I experimented with Gatorade, Fresca, Mexican Sprite, root beer, orange sodas, Coke, Diet Coke—in bottle form as well as in cans. I had super-cooled success with them all!

Removing the pressure very slowly from the bottle can keep the soda liquefied and give you the choice opportunity to play with super-cooled soda outside of the bottle.

Well, there you have it! That's how to freeze soda instantly. If you're not a soda drinker, you can do this same trick with water!

What Is a Candy Cannon?

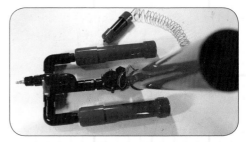

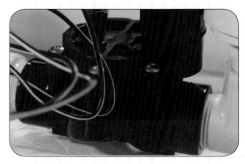

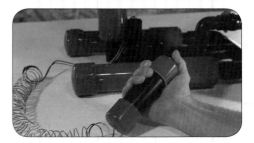

Be the coolest person on the block by building a pneumatic device that will launch candy 100 feet in the air and make it rain down all kinds of sugary treats!

It's fun to make and a huge hit at birthday parties!

WARNING:

This project uses compressed air as the medium for projecting candy, and thereby poses various safety risks. This project should not be attempted without adult supervision and adequate training. Misuse or careless use of tools or projects may result in serious injury or death. Use at your own risk.

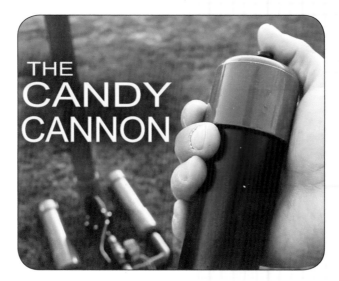

THE
CANDY
CANNON

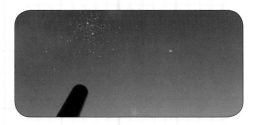

This is the Candy Cannon! It uses an electrically-activated in-line sprinkler valve rated at 150 PSI as the trigger mechanism to release compressed air through the barrel.

Just charge the system up to around 150 PSI and press the detonator button to make it fire! I built this one for my son's third birthday party to propel a payload of candy to an altitude of around 100 feet, at which point the candy begins to spread out into a giant cloud of sugary treats and drop back down, making it rain candy!

You can probably imagine the excitement of the kids with their little treat bags running all around the yard on a candy treasure hunt!

Step 1: Materials You'll Need

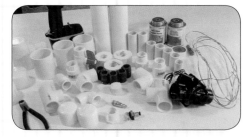

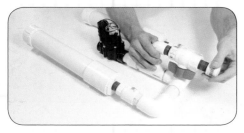

I used PVC sprinkler parts, as well as some doorbell wire, thread tape, a pneumatic adapter, and a push-button switch. Without listing individual parts, I hope the picture gives enough of an idea for you to duplicate the project.

I used 2" schedule 40 PVC pipe for the air tanks and 1" schedule 40 PVC pipe for everything else. You should be able to find all these materials at a home improvement store or sprinkler supply company.

Aside from those, you'll probably want a ¾" manual ball valve, and some other ¾" fittings that will allow you to join it to the frame.

You'll also need a 1" FIPT in-line sprinkler valve.

To make the air tanks, cut two sections of the 2" PVC pipes 12" long.

Cut your 1" pipe to custom lengths (Anywhere from 2"–4"). Feel free to use some creativity to modify the system, but basically it will look like this when the pieces are dry-fit together.

The system is designed to accept compressed air through a pneumatic adaptor we'll add to the cap near the manual ball valve. This valve allows you to close off the system, and the cannon will stay pressurized even if you disconnect from your source of compressed air.

A 9v battery will be used to activate the sprinkler valve. The valve is actually rated at 24 volts, but I've found a single 9v seems to work for this purpose.

If you're happy with how the pieces fit together, then it's time to make it permanent by cementing it together!

By the way, did you notice these parts strongly resemble the parts I used in my Rocket Rifle project?

Step 2: Make It Permanent

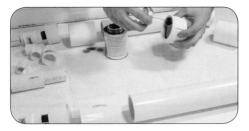

To cement PVC properly, you'll need some purple primer and some PVC cement. Some brands of PVC cement are self priming. An example would be something like Christy's Red Hot Blue Glue.

Make sure to read the instructions carefully on both the can of primer and can of PVC cement. There are dangers associated with each, and attention to detail is required in order to get a good connection that can withstand 150 PSI. Remember, this system is going to be containing a dangerous amount of pressure, so you'll want to do it right the first time!

Prime all the parts that will be in contact, and when they are dry, cement it up as instructed on the can.

Step 3: Cannon Wads

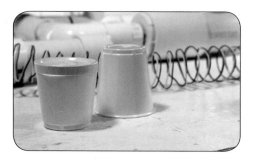

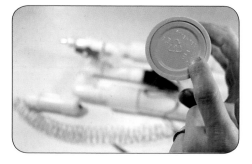

To make sure the candy launches efficiently, you may want to make a basic cannon wad from two plastic cups.

I cut ¼" off the top of a small three-ounce plastic cup and cut the bottom part off a regular sized cup then I fit them together to make this little container. This design had impressive structural integrity, which meant it could withstand the blasts of high air pressure, and be used multiple times before having to make a new one. The diameter of the wad is about as perfect as I could find for the inside of the 2" candy barrel.

You may also notice a coil of wire in the background of the picture. This is doorbell wire that connects the valve to the detonator button. I wrapped the wire around a length of the 1" pipe to form the coil.

Step 4: Finishing Touches

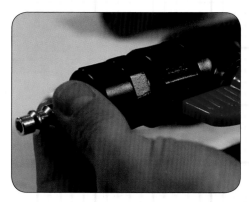

Here you can see where the pneumatic adaptor is attached, and if you like, you can give your system a paint job like I did here. I chose red and black spray paint for mine.

The pneumatic adapter is where an air hose can be connected to charge it up, and the manual ball valve gives the option of closing off the system. This means the system could maintain pressure even while the air hose was disconnected, thus making it portable.

If you don't have an air compressor, you could change out the pneumatic adaptor with a valve stem to be used with a bike pump.

Step 5: Making It Work!

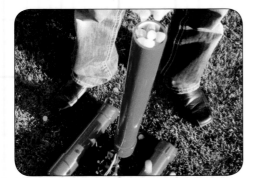

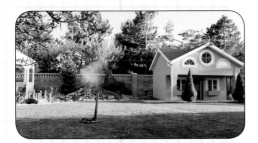

The wad goes in first and is pushed to the bottom with a ramrod, and then candy gets inserted. I used a big bag of jelly candies for practice.

Individually wrapped candies are a better choice when actually using for a party. However, these jelly candies were mainly for testing the ballistics of small, dense candies.

When the detonator button is pressed, the sprinkler valve opens and blasts the cannon wad upward. The wad pushes all the candy out with a considerable force. In this case, three pounds of candy was launched up around 100 feet in the air!

This has become a hit at birthday parties, and we are making it a tradition to do a candy launch at each of our kids' birthdays. And, of course, the birthday boy is the one who gets to push the detonator button!

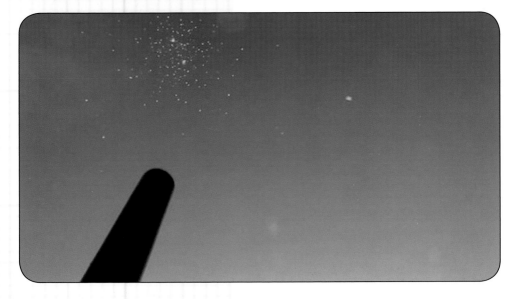

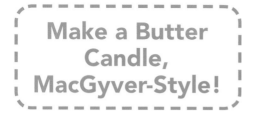

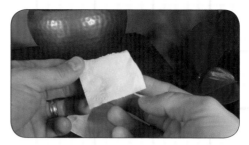

Make a Butter Candle, MacGyver-Style!

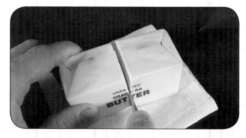

MacGyver Style
BUTTER CANDLE

Most people wouldn't think of butter as a flammable substance, but in this project it is! We're making emergency candles that burn for hours using some toilet paper and a bit of butter.

WARNING:

An open-flame poses a fire hazard. Do not use near any flammable or explosive material. Use of this content is at your own risk.

Step 1: Materials You'll Need

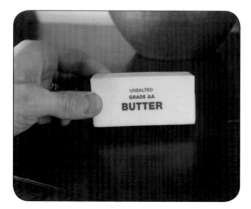

This is about as simple as it gets:
- Butter
- Toilet paper
- Something to poke a hole

Just find some butter (margarine will probably work as well) and a small piece of toilet paper. Paper towel will also work fine.

Step 2: Prepare Your Materials

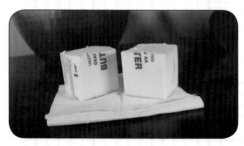

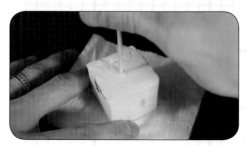

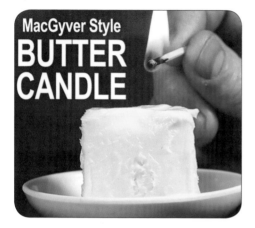

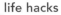

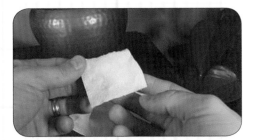

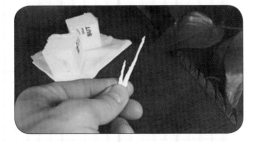

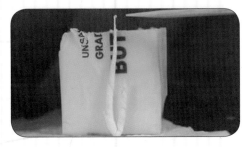

Next, take your piece of toilet paper and twist it tightly.

I put a bend at the bottom so that when it stands next to the block of butter, only about ¼" is exposed at the top.

Your butter candle is now ready for assembly.

Step 3: Wick

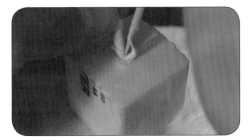

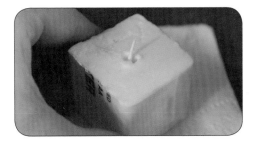

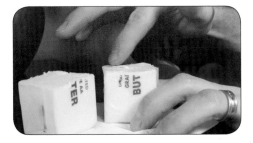

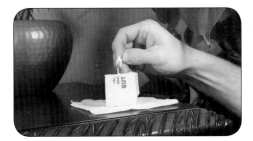

You can cut the block of butter into as many pieces as you want. As a rule of thumb, I've found that one tablespoon of butter will burn for about one hour. I used a four ounce bar of butter (eight tablespoons) and cut it in half to give me two four-hour candles (four tablespoons each).

Cutting the bar with the seam at the top will help minimize the paper from ripping as you cut through the block. Also, the colder/firmer the butter is, the cleaner your cut will be.

If you're using the same materials you should have two halves with the exposed butter side facing upward.

Take something like a skewer or toothpick and poke a hole in the top at the center. The hole should reach all the way to the bottom.

Using your skewer or toothpick, push the makeshift wick down into the hole until it touches the bottom. Give it a little twist to release and pull the stick back out.

If you did it right, you should only have ¼" of the wick poking out of the center.

The wick needs a little starter fuel, which can be added by rubbing the wick tip down into the exposed butter at the top.

Time to light it!

When you strike your match, hold the flame near the butter at the base of the wick. The butter needs to melt a little for the flame to become self-sustaining, so it may take a couple of seconds.

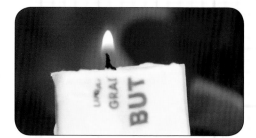

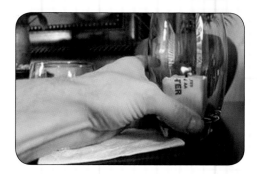

Step 4: We Have Light!

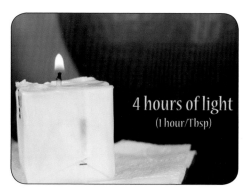

4 hours of light
(1 hour/Tbsp)

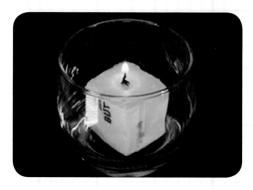

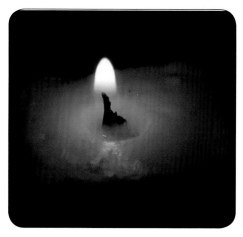

You may see the flame dim down for a few seconds at the beginning, but once the butter warms up a little, the flame should grow right back up to full size.

This works for the same reason a candle does. As the butter melts, it's wicked up into the toilet paper stem and vaporized by the heat. The vapor is flammable, and it's acting as the fuel for the flame.

These butter candles burned for four hours each, giving a total of eight hours of heat and light from the original bar.

NOTE:

After a couple of hours, the butter warms up to the point where it melts and the wick may fall over. In this case, it's useful to take a paperclip and make a support for the wick. To do this from the beginning, just insert the wick and paperclip together from the bottom of the butter block.

Dropping the candles down into something like a glass can help protect them from drafts and reduce the risk of your candle becoming a fire hazard. You also have the added benefit of an interesting DIY ambiance to your room.

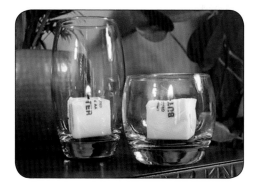

Well, now you know how to make a simple emergency candle with some toilet paper and a bit of butter!

Fight Club Soap (Bacon and Drain Cleaner Soap)!

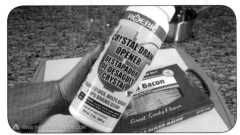

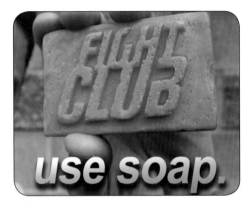

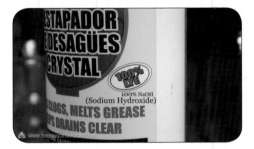

Bacon + Drain Cleaner = Soap? Yes, and it smells like cinnamon.

Project inspired by: Fight Club

Special thanks to SoapCalc.net for use of their online soap making calculator.

WARNING:

Use at own risk. Sodium Hydroxide (NaOH) is highly caustic, poisonous, and can cause serious damage to tissue and/or property. Lye should be approached with care and caution, ensuring all suggestions listed on the container are complied with and handled with gloves or other protection. There are risks associated with these projects that require adult supervision.

Step 1: Two Main Ingredients

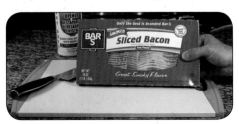

For this project I tried making traditional lye soap, which consists of two main ingredients—animal fats and lye (sodium hydroxide).

I practiced with rendering beef fat to extract "tallow," and after a few successful attempts at making soap, I wondered if it could be done with bacon fat.

To give this project a bit of a twist, I tried using one pound of "American-style" bacon because it's very fatty, and some crystal drain opener marked as 100 percent lye. It's very important that this is 100 percent lye, and if there are any doubts, it shouldn't be used. The goal here is 100 percent sodium hydroxide, which this container is, according to the Material Safety Data Sheet (MSDS).

Step 2: Render the Fat

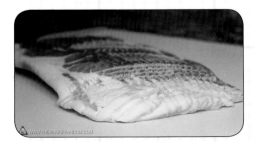

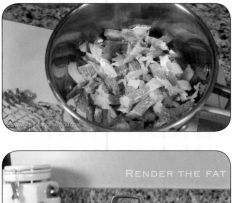

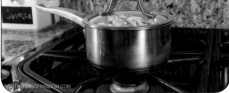

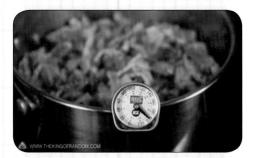

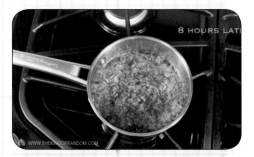

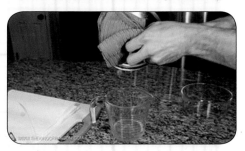

Bacon is salty and odorous, and to extract the pure fat, we need to render it.

This is best achieved by cutting the bacon into very small pieces and placing in a pot with a lid on low heat. To get clean, white fat, make sure you simmer on a very low heat—the lower the heat, the better. Higher temperatures will cause the fat to turn brown and retain some of the smell. Yes, it will take longer to extract the fat on low temps, but the quality will be worth it.

I found that a temperature of around 95°C (203°F) was enough to melt the fat and keep it nice and clean.

After about eight hours of simmering, the bacon should look cooked, and your house will smell delicious.

I used the lid as a strainer to pour the fat into a container, but this crude method does allow some impurities to pass through. To "clarify" the fat, just pour a bit of water in the container, and watch the mixture separate into two different layers. The clarified fat floats on the top, while the water and impurities sink to the bottom.

From here, it's easy to cool the mix in the fridge and skim the fat from the top.

What you're left with is a beautiful, food-grade ball of lard!

From this pack of bacon, I recovered seventy grams of rendered and clarified lard. Perfect for a single bar of soap!

Step 3: The Recipe

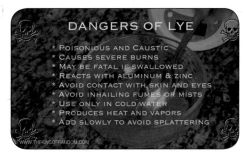

DANGERS OF LYE

* POISONOUS AND CAUSTIC
* CAUSES SEVERE BURNS
* MAY BE FATAL IF SWALLOWED
* REACTS WITH ALUMINUM & ZINC
* AVOID CONTACT WITH SKIN AND EYES
* AVOID INHAILING FUMES OR MISTS
* USE ONLY IN COLD WATER
* PRODUCES HEAT AND VAPORS
* ADD SLOWLY TO AVOID SPLATTERING

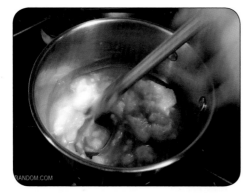

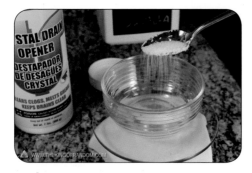

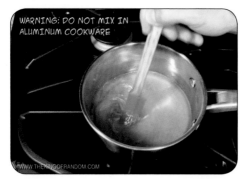

online soap-making calculator. For 70 grams of pork lard, the recipe called for 26 grams of distilled water and nine grams of sodium hydroxide. The pork lard went in a clean pot and started melting on low heat, while the water and NaOH were mixed together.

NOTE:

When working with Sodium Hydroxide, be mindful of all the risks and dangers associated with this chemical, because there are many! (See "Dangers of Lye" picture for examples)

With the lard melted, the lye solution was carefully poured in and stirred constantly on low heat for five minutes, then left to sit for five minutes more. Every five minutes after that, I came back and stirred for two minutes, then let sit for another five. This was repeated until the mixture had the consistency of vanilla pudding, and when dripped on itself, it would leave blobs and ridges. This stage of the mix is called "trace."

Step 4: Saponification

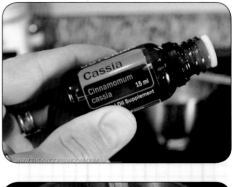

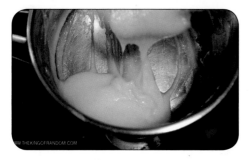

To figure out the best recipe for traditional lye soap using pork lard, I visited SoapCalc.net for use of their

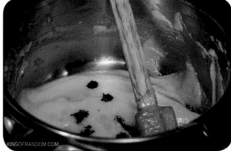

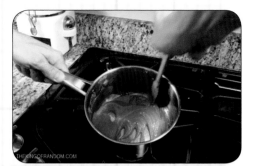

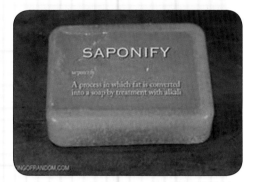

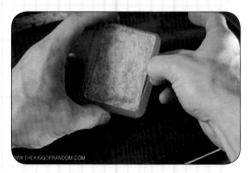

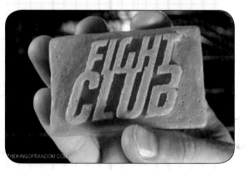

be nice and white and there should hardly be any smell of bacon at all. For aroma, I chose to use seven drops of "Cassia" essential oil (smells like cinnamon).

For color, I used seven drops of red food coloring. For making soaps, food coloring probably isn't recommended, but it worked great for this purpose.

When the mix was stirred together, it all turned a bright pink and was ready for casting. I had fashioned a small silicone mold for the bar of soap I wanted, and poured the mix in to let it cure.

The curing process is called "saponification," which basically means the fats and alkaline solution are combining to form soap. To help speed the process, I placed the soap mold in an oven with the door closed for 24–48 hours. The heat from the oven light is enough to help the saponification take place much quicker, and firm up the bar. You can see that when the bar was removed, it had nicely taken the shape of the mold.

NOTE:

The bubbles in the soap were caused by a mistake on my part. I pre-heated the oven to 338°F (170°C) before adding the soap, and this much heat deformed the bar with bubbles. Do not pre-heat the oven at all, and your bar should come out clean and smooth.

Step 5: Getting the Bar Ready for Use

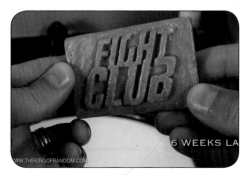

6 WEEKS LA

At the "trace" stage, aromas and colors could be added to make the bar a little more attractive if desired. If the lard was rendered properly, it should

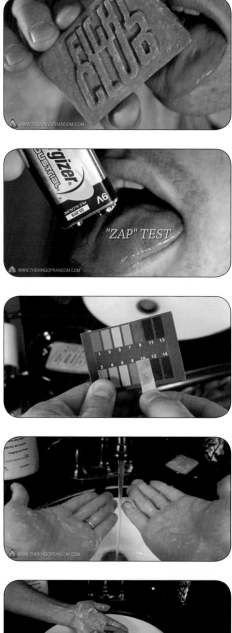

Before you use your bar of soap, you need to make sure it's fully saponified or else the lye in the bar can burn your skin.

The easiest way to tell if the bar is ready is to lick it. If it tastes like a bar of soap, it is. On the other hand, if it zaps you like licking a nine-volt battery, it needs more time to cure.

I let my bar cure for six weeks just to be safe. The result was a much firmer bar that holds up substantially longer in the shower and was richer in color.

I tested the pH value with litmus paper and got a value somewhere around 7.5. Anywhere between seven and ten should be fine for your soaps.

Washing my hands, you can see the soap bubbles like you'd expect. If you want more of a lather, there are other oils you can add for different effects like hardness, lather, cleansing, etc. Soapcalc.net should have plenty of info if you search around.

This is glycerin soap, meaning the glycerin was left in the bar. Most manufacturers extract the glycerin out of the soap to resell as a different product. So in a way, this soap may be superior to many soaps bought at the store.

The glycerin helps moisturize and soften the skin. I personally tested these bars in the shower over a period of two months. They retained their cinnamon scent and color and did a good job cleaning the body.

Not surprisingly, they work just like soap!

Step 6: Bacon Bits

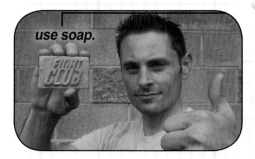

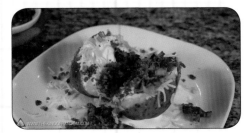

Remember the leftover bacon in the pot? Try using it to make fresh homemade bacon bits! We used these ones for dinner on our baked potatoes!

Well, now you know how to make a beautiful bar of glycerin soap from household drain cleaner and a pack of bacon.

Section 3
Special-Occasion Hacks

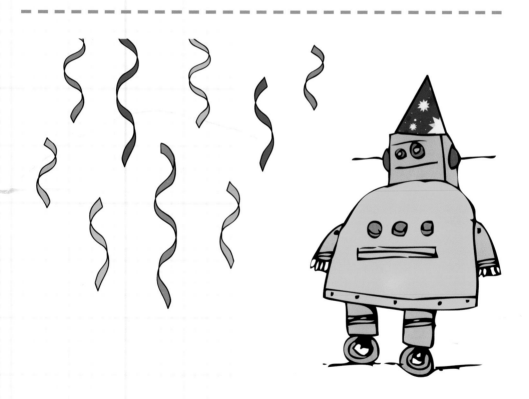

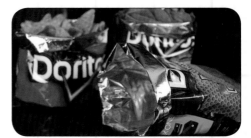

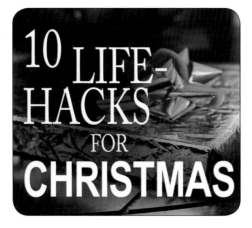

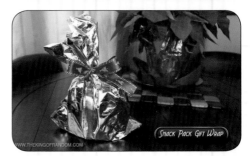

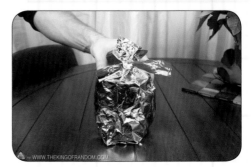

Snack Pack Gift Wrap

WWW.THEKINGOFRANDOM.COM

Ten amazing tips and tricks, for Holiday challenges!

In this project, you'll see how to:

• Convert a bag of chips into decorative wrapping paper.
• Protect your wrapping paper from unraveling in storage.
• Send Christmas letters without having to buy envelopes.
• Make custom festive pancakes in any shape.
• Avoid the challenges of packing tape sticking to itself.
• Make your house smell like fresh-cut pine.
• Decorate sugar cookies with no mess to clean up.
• Prevent your Christmas lights from tangling in storage.
• Make custom chocolate garnishes for entertaining.
• Turn your Christmas morning garbage into custom cards.

If you're in need of a last minute gift idea, check this out:

Grab an empty bag of chips and search around the house for something you think could work as a gift.

Clean the chip bag and turn it inside out, then carefully place your gift inside and twist the bag at the top.

All you need to do now is grab a ribbon, tie a bow, and your instant gift is ready to go.

Now, if you don't have a ribbon handy, it's no problem. Just cut the top inch off the chip bag and tie that on instead. It should be just enough to get you by in your time of need.

Paper Keeper

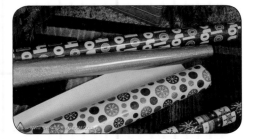

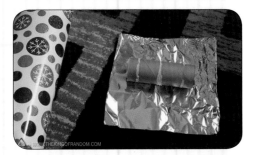

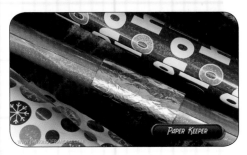

Better Letters

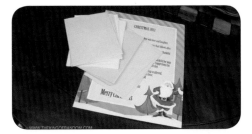

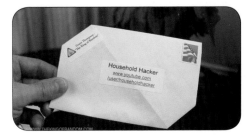

With internet and email becoming so common, you may not have any envelopes to send out Christmas letters.

Rather than going out and buying some, just take your letter and crease it in the center, then fold opposite corners into the center line.

Fold the two edges next, and then with a slight turn, the tips are folded in to complete a rectangle.

When you tuck these two corners into the flaps underneath them, your letter has just transformed into its own envelope.

All you need to do now is address it, add a stamp, and your letter is ready for posting.

If you've got rolls of wrapping paper that you want preserved, head to the kitchen and finish up some leftovers so you can salvage the aluminum foil.

Now cut the foil into a square that's a couple inches longer than a toilet paper tube.

Next you'll need to make a cut down the side of the toilet tube, so you can wrap the foil around the outside, and fold the edges inward to hold it in place.

Push the foil in at the ends and now you've got a decorative clasp that will clamp around your tube and hold your wrapping paper in place.

Your decorative wrap is preserved for another year.

Posh Pancakes

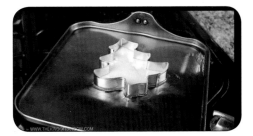

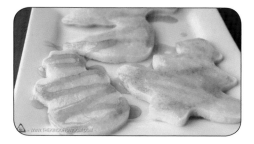

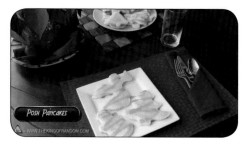

To make a fun and festive breakfast, start by pouring your pancake mix into a cleaned-out condiment bottle.

Now, dip some large metal cookie cutters into a small tray of cooking oil and set it on a pre-greased and pre-heated cooking pan.

Now just pour in some pancake batter and give it a minute to cook.

When the batter is firm, go ahead and remove the cookie cutter with a clean pair of pliers, and your pancake will hold its shape.

Now just finish them up in the usual way, and then make a whole bunch more.

Add some butter and a drizzle of maple syrup, and you've got a festive and impressive holiday breakfast.

Grab Tab

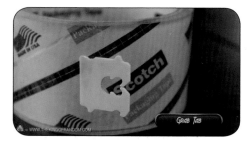

When you're wrapping packages, you know the frustration that comes when you can't find the edge of the tape. And when you do find it, it's surprisingly difficult to get it up. The solution is a simple bread clip.

There's a good chance you have one of these lying around, and all you need to do is just tuck it under the edge of the tape.

This custom "grab tab" will save your spot without damaging the tape at all, and makes a nice little handle for pulling the tape up when you need it.

If you don't have a bread clip, try using a penny instead.

Air Care

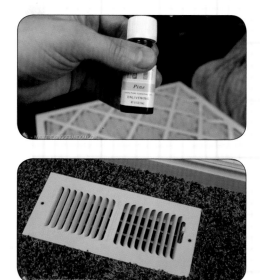

Your Christmas tree may be fake, but you can still enjoy the scent of a fresh-cut tree.

Just take the air filter from your furnace and pick up a bottle of pine essential oil.

And remember that a little goes a long way.

Now add 10–20 drops on the backside of the filter, and then place it back into position.

Open up your air register, sit back, and enjoy the fresh piney aroma.

Nicer Cookie Icer

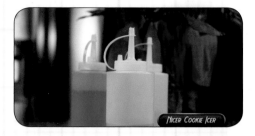

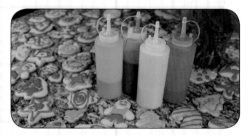

When the cookies are baked and ready for frosting, it can be a pretty messy job. And no matter how hard you try, they still look like they were frosted by a four-year-old. You can win this challenge by pouring your frosting into a few different condiment containers.

Screw the caps on tight, and now you've got a much nicer cookie icer.

This will give you so much decorating precision that your imagination is the only limitation.

There's no sugary mess to clean up, and if you press the cap back on, your frosting will stay good for days.

Light Saver

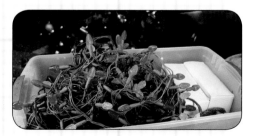

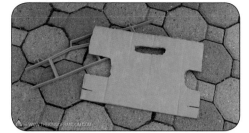

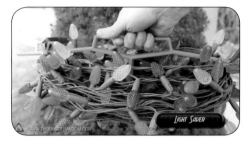

When the season's over and it's time to take the Christmas lights down, you know that throwing them in a bin just means you'll have a major rat's nest to deal with next year.

Try using a simple extension cord holder instead. You can find these at hardware stores for about a dollar and a half.

When your lights are wrapped, plug the two ends of the cord together, and now you're guaranteed to be tangle free.

By the way, if you can't find one of these cord wrappers, try making one out of a piece of cardboard. It will work just as well, and nothing beats the price of free.

Shavings for Cravings

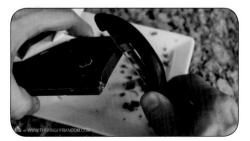

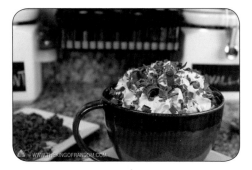

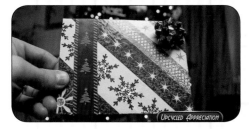

When you're entertaining friends with a nice warm chocolaty drink, go one step farther by grabbing a potato peeler and their favorite chocolate bar.

Carefully shave down the side of the candy bar, and you'll see it creates a decorative chocolate garnishing.

You can use these tasty shavings to deliciously garnish their drink or decorate anything else you can think of.

Your friends will be super impressed and wonder why they never thought of this.

Up-Cycled Appreciation

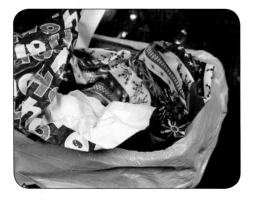

Rather than letting all that wrapping paper go to waste, try removing little decorations, like ribbons and bows, and then use glue or spray adhesive to attach the wrapping paper back to the box your present came in.

Now, cut a rectangle about the size of a postcard and reattach the bows and ribbons.

Just like that, you've got an impressive "thank you" card to return your appreciation.

Your family and friends will be blown away, and hey, it's better for the environment anyway.

In Closing

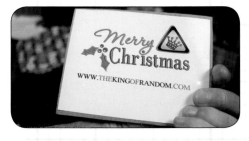

Well, there are a few ideas that will hopefully make your Christmas a little merrier.

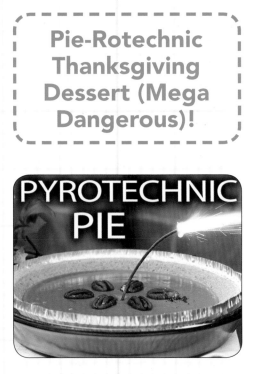

An innocent-looking pumpkin pie erupts in an insane fountain of flames and fire!

WARNING:

This project is for demonstrational, educational, and entertainment purposes only. It is not intended to be duplicated. This experiment should only be attempted by experienced professionals. Use of content is at own risk.

Disclaimer

Walking through the bakery at the grocery store the other day, I took a close look at the pumpkin pies on display. They made me realize how similar "R-candy" and pumpkin pie are in appearance. That got the wheels spinning and spawned this video.

NOTE:

This is for entertainment purposes only, and isn't intended to be duplicated.

However, having said that, here's how I made it.

Step 1: Composition

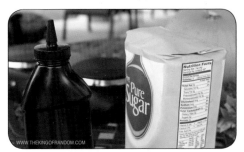

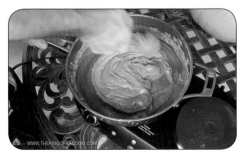

The "pie filling" composition is nothing more than a 60 percent/40 percent mix by weight of KNO3 and sugar.

I used a digital scale to measure the ingredients together, and then shook them together in a large mixing bowl to ensure uniform composition.

The mixture was cooked on medium heat, while stirring as often as was required until the mix became light-brown in color and the consistency of pie filling.

Step 2: Setting Up

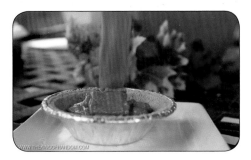

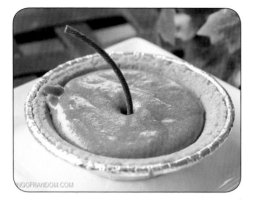

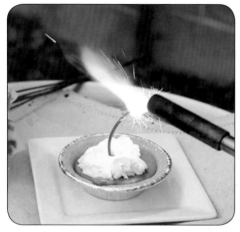

Step 3: Ignition

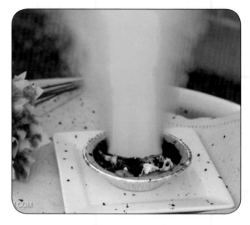

You can see in the picture that the pie erupts like a volcano, spewing molten fuel up and out.

The small pies burn violently for about 15–20 seconds.

Step 4: Go Bigger!

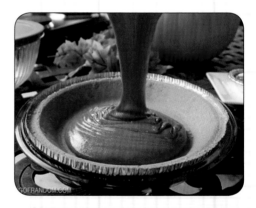

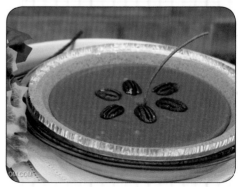

When the R-candy mix was the right consistency, I poured it into a small pie crust.

Five minutes later, I inserted a fuse for convenience in igniting the mix. I chose five minutes, because any sooner, and the fuse will fall over into the mix, and any later, and you run the risk of the composition setting up as firm as hard candy. After that, nothing will go in unless you drill a hole.

Finally, I added whipping cream around the top. This served two purposes:

• It makes it look even more like a pie.
• It added a layer of protection from the burning fuse embers. Without this layer, the pie can ignite prematurely and at unpredictable spots due to the spray of burning embers.

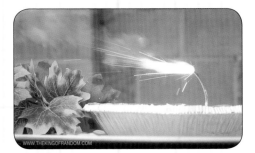

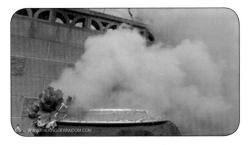

It takes a considerable amount of composition to fill a large pie crust, which means a lot more stored energy waiting to be released!

One Facebook fan said that this is the pie that "burns its own calories." I agree!

Step 5: Slightly Overcooked?

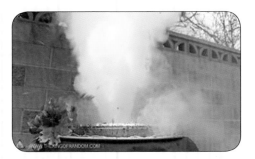

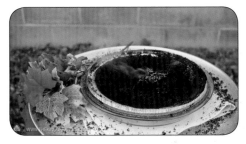

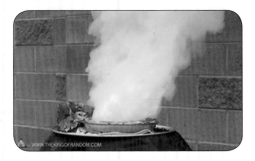

It's worth mentioning that although one of the main ingredients is sugar, the fuel is not edible.

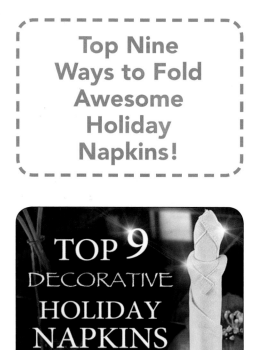

WARNING:

Dinner guests may become overly intimidated by your amazing napkin folding skills. Use of content is at own risk.

In this project, I decided to play with the art of napkin-folding, and these are the nine that I liked the most for this holiday season.

Fancy Napkin #1: The "Crown"

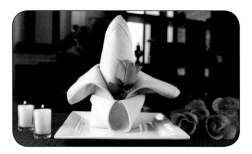

Making the "Crown" is as simple as following eight easy steps.

1. Lay out a square napkin and begin by folding it up diagonally to form a triangle.
2. Fold up each of the bottom corners to meet the point at the top. If your napkin isn't perfectly square, just do the best you can with what you have.
3. Now fold the bottom point three quarters of the way up.
4. After this, fold it back on itself so the point is back at the bottom.
5. Go ahead and flip it over.
6. Take one of the back edges and fold it a third of the way in.
7. The other side folds over next and is secured by tucking the corner into the flap at the bottom.
8. Flip it over one more time and now just peel the two sides down like you're peeling a banana.
9. Open the base, stand it upright, and your cloth crown is finished.

This simple fold is quick and easy, and can add a very elegant touch to your table settings.

If you don't have any cloth napkins, try using paper napkins instead.

Fancy Holiday Napkin #2: The "Candle"

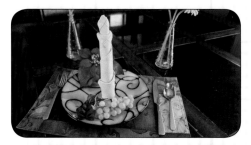

To fold the candle, we're going to follow eight simple steps.

1. Start with a square napkin and turn it slightly so that one point is facing up.
2. Now take the bottom tip and fold it up toward the top until the two

corners match. This should form a rough triangle.

3. The next step is to fold the base up just a couple of inches and press it down flat.
4. At this point, we can flip the whole thing over so the triangle is pointing to the left.
5. Take the bottom point and fold it up so the tip is just past the center.
6. Start rolling the whole thing into a tube, starting from the bottom and working toward the top. When your roll is finished, you might want to push the uneven ends back into the tube, and then tuck the loose end neatly into the cuff. This should give you a nice sturdy base to hold your napkin upright.
7. To finish off, just turn one layer of the tip down.
8. After this, shape the other layer to look like a flame.

Now your candle looks like it's burning with a bit of wax dripping off the top. It's completely finished and ready to impress.

Now, if you don't have cloth napkins, try making this with a paper napkin instead. It works just as well as long as you're gentle and careful not to tear the paper.

Fancy Napkin #3: Simple "Silverware Pouch"

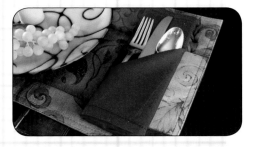

We can make a fancy silverware pouch in just six easy steps:
1. Start at the bottom of a square napkin and fold the two corners up so the edges line up at the top.

2. Now take the right side and fold the napkin in half again to form a square.
3. Fold the top left corner of the top layer down to the opposite side.
4. Go ahead and flip the whole thing over.
5. Fold the right side a third of the way in.
6. After that, fold the left edge back over top and tuck the bottom corner down inside the pocket on the other.

When it's flipped right-side-up, you can see the pouch is completely finished, so just add some silverware and set it out to impress.

Of course, if you don't have any cloth napkins, these folds will work just as well with paper napkins and plastic utensils.

Fancy Napkin #4: The "Pyramid"

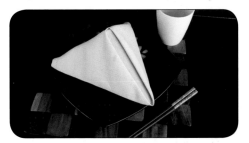

The "Pyramid" is simple, and can be done in just six easy steps:
1. Lay out a square napkin and begin by folding it up diagonally to form a triangle.
2. Fold up one of the bottom corners to meet the point at the top.
3. Do the same thing with the point on the other side.
4. Flip the whole thing over.
5. Now just fold it in half from the top to the bottom.
6. Lift it from the center so that it folds in on itself.

When you stand it upright, your decorative napkin pyramid is finished.

You can probably guess that this will work with paper napkins as well.

Fancy Napkin #5: The "Elf Shoe"

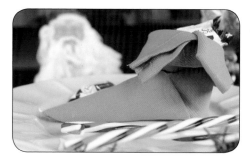

We can make the "Elf Shoe" in eight fairly simple steps:

1. Fold a square napkin in half from the bottom to the top.
2. After that, fold it again from the top to the bottom.
3. Now find the center and fold the two sides in the same way you'd fold a paper airplane.
4. Go ahead and continue this idea by folding the sides in again, forming a sharp point at the tip.
5. At this point, the two halves can fold over on each other, and when you flatten them out, check which side is open and make sure it's facing to the bottom.
6. Now focus on the loose parts at the back and fold the top layer up and out of the way.
7. The bottom layer folds in half, and then wraps over the top layer, tucking neatly into the little flap in the side of the shoe.
8. All that's left now is to turn down the loose material sticking up at the top to form a little cuff.

Your little elf shoe napkin is finished and ready for showing off. If you try making one out of a paper napkin, it will probably look something like this.

Fancy Napkin #6: The "Basket"

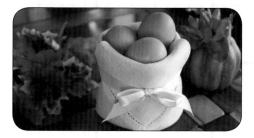

To make the "Basket," we're going to follow seven steps:

1. First, fold a square napkin diagonally to form a triangle.
2. Fold the base up about three or four inches from the bottom.
3. Now flip the whole thing over so the triangle is pointing to the left.
4. Take the top point and fold it down so it's just short of the bottom by a couple of inches.
5. Fold the bottom point a few inches past the top edge and tuck it around the backside of the pouch.
6. Fold the point of the top layer down over the front of the pouch.
7. Fold the back layer down over the back side.

Go ahead and straighten up the edges, fluff up the pouch a bit, and your basket is finished.

If you tie a ribbon around the top, it adds an amazing amount of stability, and of course, the same folds will work on paper napkins as well. Now you know how to fold a decorative napkin basket.

Fancy Napkin #7: The "Rose"

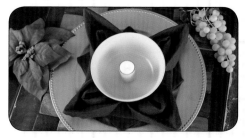

The "Rose" can be folded in just six easy steps:

1. Get started with a square napkin and fold each of the four corners into the center as best you can. Most napkins aren't perfectly square, but just do the best you can with what you've got.
2. The next step is to take the four new corners and fold them into the center as well.
3. Now just hold everything together at the middle and flip the napkin over.
4. Let's repeat the process again by taking these four corners and folding them into the middle like we did the others.
5. Okay, we're just about done, so to finish up, hold the center firmly with one hand and gently pull the tips from underneath the corners until they look like flower petals.
6. When you've done this to each of the four corners, do the same thing to the undersides of the edges. This will make little points stick out between your rose petals and give the whole thing a nice symmetrical balance.

This adds an amazing decorative flare to your dinner presentation, and if you don't have any cloth napkins, these can look great with paper napkins as well.

Fancy Napkin #8: "Bird of Paradise"

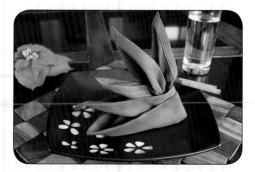

To make the "Bird of Paradise," we're going to follow eight simple steps:

1. To get started, fold a square napkin into quarters and turn it so the open ends are pointing away from you.
2. Now fold the bottom end up to the top so it forms a triangle.
3. Flip the whole thing over.
4. Next we'll need to fold the two sides in so they meet in the middle, which should be easy to do if you think of folding a paper airplane.
5. When the two sides are flattened out, flip it over again.
6. Fold the two triangular tabs at the back in toward the center.
7. Now just fold the triangle in half lengthwise and cradle it in your hand so that the open ends are facing into your palm.
8. Go ahead and peel back each of the four layers inside, and when they're spaced the way you want them, your fancy napkin is ready to dazzle.

This looks awesome with a cloth napkin, but I found you can make it with a paper napkin as well. Just be gentle when you pull the layers apart so they don't rip.

Fancy Napkin #9: The "Bishop's Hat"

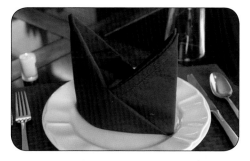

We can make the Bishop's Hat in eight easy steps:

1. Start by folding a square napkin in half from top to bottom and crease it in the middle.

2. Now fold the bottom left corner up to the middle of the top edge.
3. Fold the top right corner to the middle of the bottom edge.
4. Go ahead and flip it over.
5. Fold one of the edges up to meet the other, and then pull the point out from under the top fold.
6. To finish up, just crease the left side triangle in half and tuck it into the fold of the other.
7. Now flip it over again.
8. Repeat the same thing on the other side, and when that's tucked into place, gently pull the napkin open at the bottom and set it upright.

You can see these are simple to make, and setting them on your dinner plates adds a dash of class.

Secret Napkin

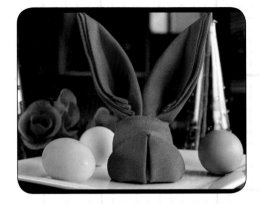

Well, now you know how to fold nine different decorative napkins for the holiday season, so go out and impress someone!

How to Make an Exploding Pumpkin Face (Blast-O-Lantern)

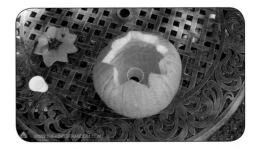

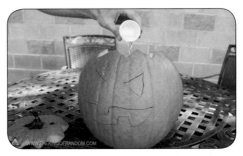

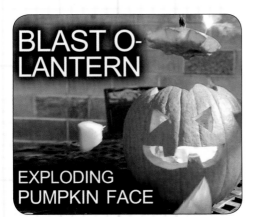

Exploding Pumpkin Faces! You could try making them this Halloween, but probably shouldn't. Happy Halloween!

WARNING:

This project is for demonstrational, educational, and entertainment purposes only. It is not intended to be duplicated. CaC2 mixed with water produces acetylene gas, which, when mixed with oxygen, creates an extremely flammable gas.

Step 1: Forming the Gas

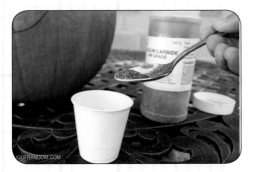

A very flammable gas (acetylene) is produced inside a pre-carved pumpkin shell by mixing CaC2 and water. When the gas is ignited, the pressure inside builds rapidly, forcing the carved pieces to blast out dramatically.

Step 2: Ignition

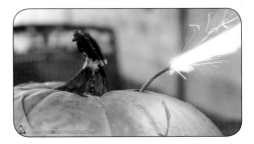

I chose to ignite the gas with a piece of Visco fuse. I found it actually ignites most consistently with a hole just small enough to poke the fuse through, and works better at the back of the pumpkin. I only placed it at the top here so it would be visible. In reality, placing the fuse near the opening at the top leads to premature ignition more often than not, and isn't recommended.

Step 3: Exploding Pumpkin Faces

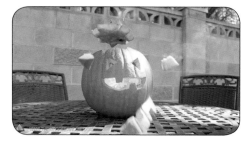

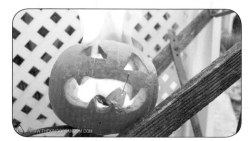

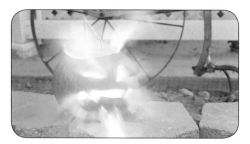

Happy Halloween!

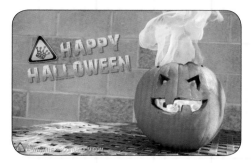

How to Make Carbonated Ice Cream, "Halloween-Style" (Dry Ice Cream)!

Dry Ice (With a Fire Extinguisher?)

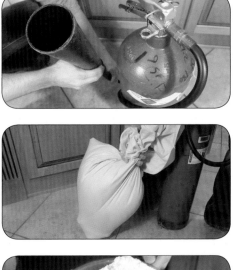

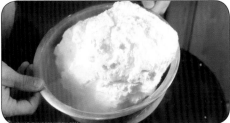

Carbonated ice cream? Really! And here's how to make it with a few simple ingredients and a bit of dry ice.

WARNING:

Dry ice is extremely cold (–78C/ –109F) and can cause instant frostbite to exposed skin. This project should not be attempted without adult supervision and adequate training. Ingestion of dry ice may cause serious internal tissue damage. If dry ice is ingested, drink copious amounts of warm water as soon as possible. Misuse or careless use may result in serious injury.

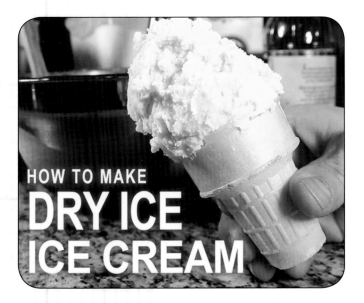

HOW TO MAKE DRY ICE ICE CREAM

how to make carbonated ice cream, "halloween-style" (dry ice cream)!

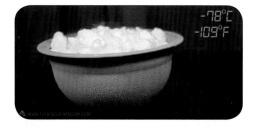

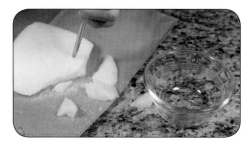

Step 1: What You'll Need

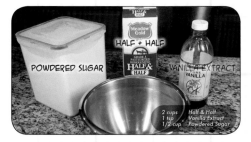

This simple vanilla ice cream recipe is easy and delicious!

- 2 cups Half & Half
- 1 tsp. vanilla extract
- 1/2 cup powdered sugar

NOTE:

Half & Half is a dairy product consisting of half light cream and half milk. If you have heavy whipping cream and milk, you can make half and half by combining four parts whole milk with one part heavy cream. If you only have light whipping cream, use three parts whole milk and one part light whipping cream.

You may remember in a previous project how we used a carbon dioxide (CO2) fire extinguisher to produce dry ice. For this project, I tried discharging the entire 15-pound extinguisher to see how much we could get, and ended up with 5 pounds of dry ice. Not bad!

Certain fire extinguishers utilize CO2 as the medium for suppressing fires. These types are mainly found in restaurant kitchens, mechanical rooms, and in areas that hold sensitive equipment like computers.

CO2 fire extinguishers are usually charged with food-grade CO2 and are referred to in terms of pounds. For example, a 5-pound CO2 extinguisher is charged with a 5-pound weight of liquid CO2. The extinguisher is then highly pressurized.

CO2 fire extinguishers are marked with stickers or holes punched in the servicing labels. They also have unusually large discharge horns and no pressure gauges.

Of course, if you don't have access to a CO2 fire extinguisher, try getting some dry ice at your local grocery store. This will work just as well (and a lot cheaper) than getting it any other way.

Step 2: Add the Cold

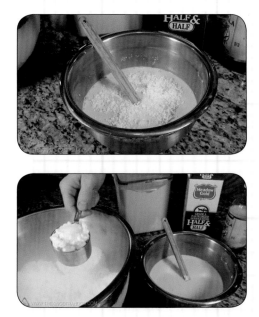

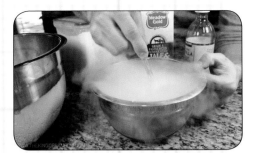

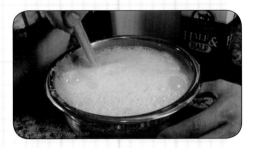

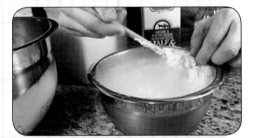

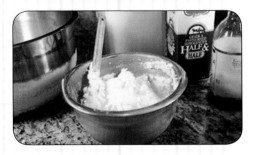

moderation, as the mix needs it. I love this method because it adds a mysterious flowing fog quality to the process that's very visually stimulating and gratifying.

When the fog stops, the dry ice has most likely all sublimated out, but be careful when eating, and watch for any small pieces that may have been missed, and avoid eating them. Because the CO_2 sublimates directly into a gas, it's very clean and doesn't leave behind any residue.

Dry ice is solid CO_2, and as it sublimates through the mix, it forms carbonic acid with some of the water in the mix, giving the ice cream the familiar fizzy carbonated taste that we associate with soda.

Step 3: Ready to Serve!

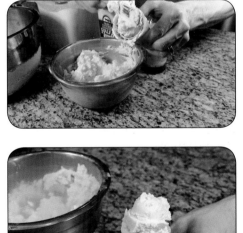

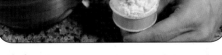

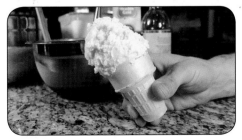

Mix all ingredients together and add dry ice. The dry ice cools the liquid mixture to the point where it takes on the familiar qualities of ice cream.

BE CAREFUL! If you add too much dry ice all at once, your ice cream mix will bubble over and spill out all over your counter. This makes a very big mess, so avoid the hassle by adding dry ice in

The ice cream should be ready when it looks and feels like, well, ice cream!

When you are convinced there are no more chunks of dry ice in the mix, and no more vapor is rising from the ice cream, it's a pretty safe bet that all the dry ice has sublimated out.

The awesome thing about using a cooling medium like dry ice is that it doesn't leave behind any watery residue in the mix. It all just vaporizes out, leaving the chilled ice cream behind. When you're sure it's safe to eat, go ahead and transfer it to a cone or a dish for serving.

Step 4: Enjoy!

You've just created a carbonated ice cream cone! That means it's slightly fizzy and will tingle your tongue a bit. When my kids got a taste of the tingly treat, they couldn't get enough.

Well, now you know how to make a delicious carbonated ice cream in a way that's appropriate for Halloween, but fun any time of the year.

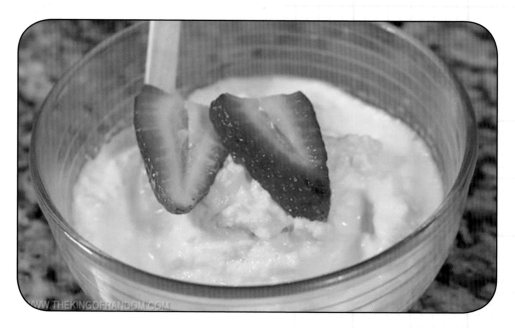

Things to Do at a Birthday Party with Liquid Nitrogen!

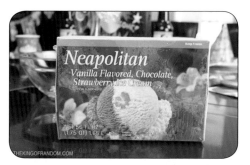

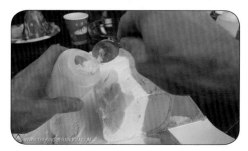

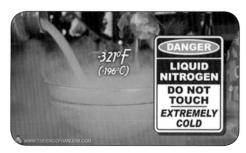

Some tricks with liquid nitrogen that you could try at your next party but probably shouldn't!

WARNING:

These projects and results are depictions of my own personal experiences, which may vary depending on location and modifications to project ideas. There may be risks associated with some of these projects that I'm not aware of. Liquid Nitrogen is −321°F and can cause severe tissue damage and serious damage after prolonged exposure. Use of this content is at your own risk.

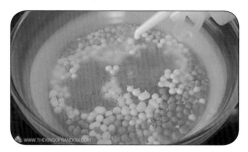

Futuristic Ice Cream (Dippin' Dots)

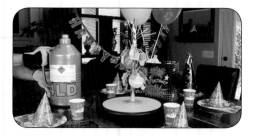

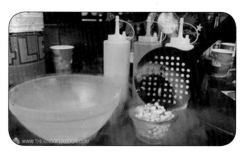

Get out your container of liquid nitrogen and grab a box of Neapolitan ice cream. This is the type of ice cream that has three flavors in one, so go ahead and separate the colors into different containers, and give them a couple of minutes to melt.

In the meantime, we'll need to fill a bowl with liquid nitrogen. This stuff is −321°F (−196°C), which means it will be well below the freezing point.

Now if you try dripping your flavors in one drop at a time, you'll notice they instantly bead up and freeze solid.

When you've got all the flavors you need, simply scoop the tasty pellets into a serving bowl and voila! You've got a futuristic ice cream ready to serve and enjoy.

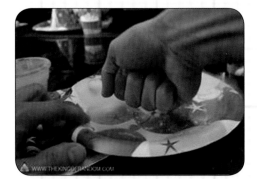

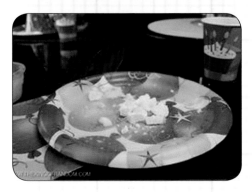

Chill Pills

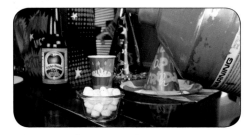

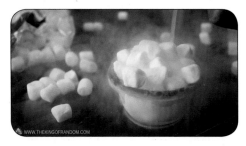

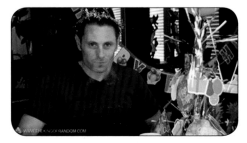

Load up a bowl with mini marshmallows, and sprinkle liquid nitrogen over the top. The marshmallows should freeze instantly, but go ahead and let them soak for about thirty seconds just to be sure.

The end result is a sub-zero "chill pill" that's perfectly fine to eat and lets you see your breath when you crunch into it.

Now if you flash-freeze a larger marshmallow, rather than eating it, try placing it on a plate and giving it a smack. It'll shatter into a thousand pieces.

Noise Makers

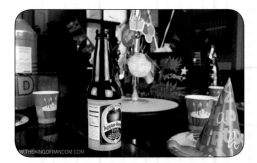

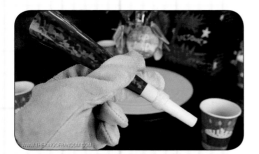

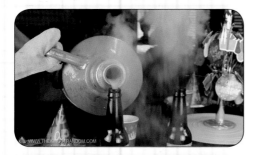

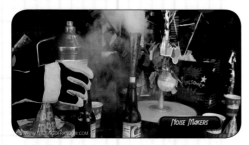

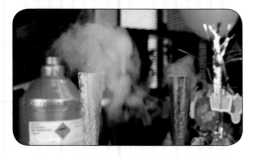

place, it becomes a crazy noisemaker that blows all on its own.

If you get a few of these going, you can really make some noise.

Balloon Blowers

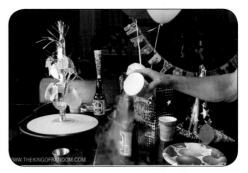

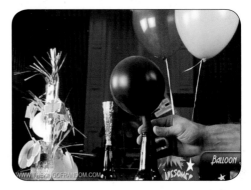

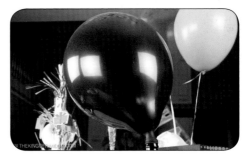

For this trick you'll need a glass bottle with a narrow neck and a party horn with a little hot glue added around the bottom. When it gets placed in the bottle, it should make a nice, snug fit.

Now carefully pour the liquid nitrogen so the bottle is a quarter full, followed by a shot of hot water. You can see that when the horn is pressed into

When there isn't enough pressure to keep the horns going, try adding more hot water to the bottle and place a balloon over the top.

There will still be enough pressure shooting up to inflate the balloons all on their own. It will save you the effort, and the gas inside is completely harmless.

Chips that "Bite Back"

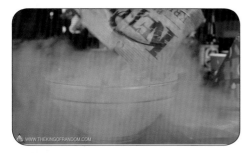

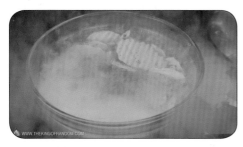

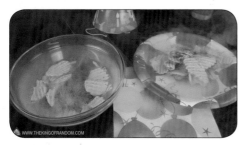

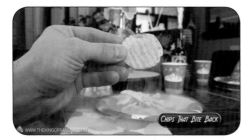

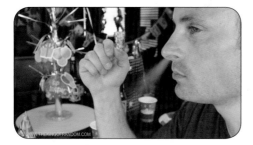

Find a bag of your favorite chips and dump them all into a bowl of liquid nitrogen to sit for a couple of minutes. Now it may look like they're boiling, but they're actually being cooled to a ridiculously low temperature. When the "boiling" stops, feel free to scoop them out and put them onto a plate for serving.

If you try eating one of these right now, you might feel a sharp sting on your tongue, like the chip is trying to bite you back. But if you give them just a minute, then try chewing with your mouth closed, it should take your chip-eating experience to a whole new level.

Liquid Oxygen

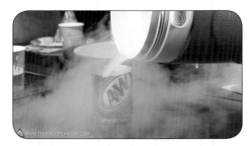

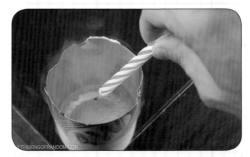

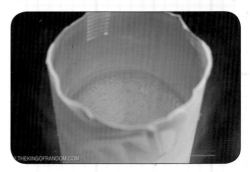

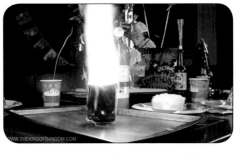

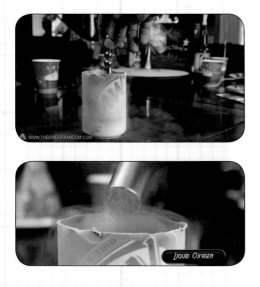

LIQUID OXYGEN

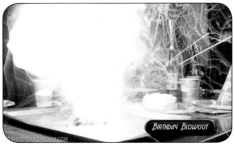

BIRTHDAY BLOWOUT

Cut the top off an empty soda can and fill it up with liquid nitrogen. You can see that holding a flame into the can will make it go out. But if you let the can sit for a few minutes, the extreme cold will pull oxygen out of the air and trap it at the bottom.

Now try dipping a super strong magnet into the liquid, and when you pull it out, you'll have liquid oxygen stuck to the bottom. At least until it warms up and boils off.

Birthday Blowout

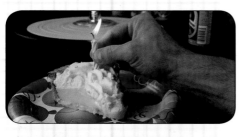

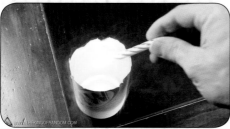

Save one of the candles from your birthday cake and hold it over the can.

You'll notice that this time the flame actually gets brighter. This is because the nitrogen has evaporated and left the oxygen behind. Pure oxygen is extremely reactive, and if you drop a candle down into the liquid, you can see it gets so hot that the metal can actually melts in just a few seconds, and then explodes, spewing molten metal all over the place.

This is a trick that should be done outside, keeping the safety of you and your guests a top priority.

Balloon Babies

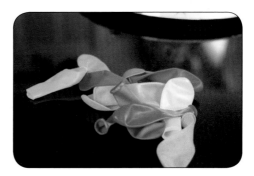

things to do at a birthday party with liquid nitrogen!

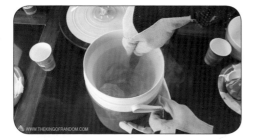

Fly Babies

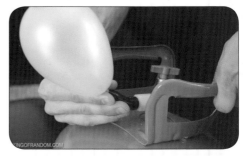

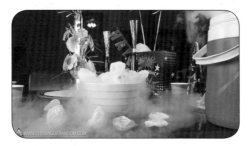

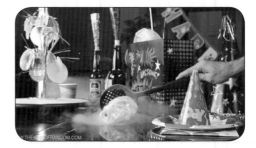

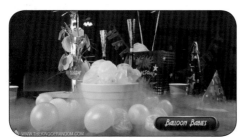

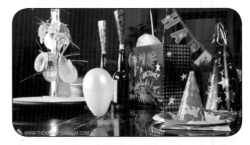

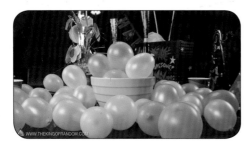

BALLOON BABIES

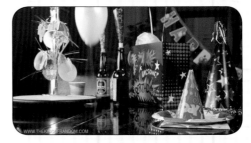

Blow up a bunch of little party balloons and soak them in a container of liquid nitrogen so they shrink down to nothing.

Then, quickly scoop them all into a bowl and stand back to watch the magic. Rising from a layer of mysterious flowing fog, your little balloon babies begin to grow right before your eyes, spilling over and covering the table.

They grow up so fast, don't they?

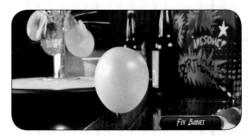

FLY BABIES

Fill one of your small balloons with helium and shrink it down in liquid nitrogen like you did the others.

Scoop it out and place it down on a table to see what happens.

You'll notice that after a few seconds, it suddenly pops upright and takes off like a little UFO.

Your friends should be impressed to see your little creation grow up, spread its wings, and begin to fly.

Kryptonian "Super Breath"

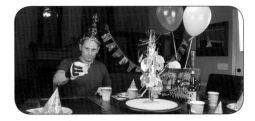

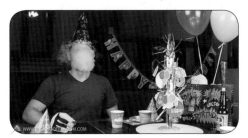

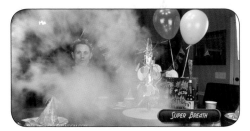

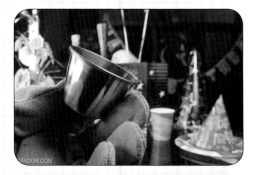

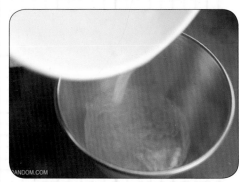

For this last trick, we'll need a shot glass or a small condiment cup. Pour in a tiny bit of liquid nitrogen and get ready to put it in your mouth.

As long as you spit it back out immediately, you'll gain the Kryptonian power of superbreath.

Just make sure not to swallow or take too long getting it back out. That probably wouldn't end well.

Section 4
Money-Saving Hacks

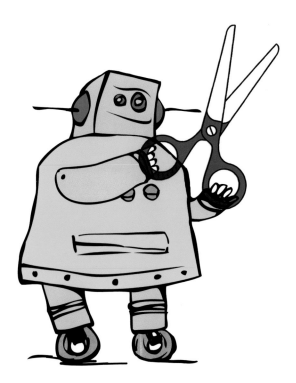

WARNING:

Extreme caution should be used when cutting into sheetrock. There may be electrical wires or other sensitive materials behind the wall that can't be seen, and could be damaged when cutting. Use of content is at own risk.

Why a Secret Safe?

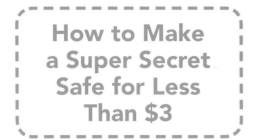

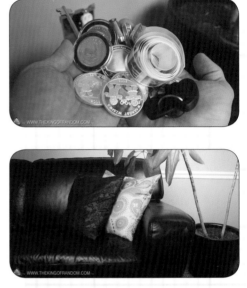

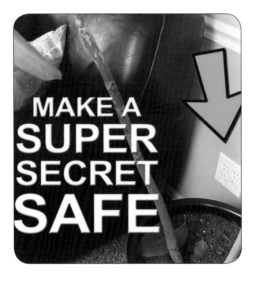

In this project you'll learn how to make a super secret safe that nobody will recognize, even if they're looking straight at it.

I saw a picture of a hidden wall safe on LifeHacker.com and found it was a product being sold for about eight dollars from ThinkGeek.com.

Rather than order one, it seemed feasible to make one with just a couple of materials from the hardware store. Not to mention, it's much cheaper.

There are so many variations that could be made to this idea. I demonstrated four that I came up with, and perhaps the best one is the box behind your cable. If you use one of those, it's completely free and you don't have to cut any new holes in your walls.

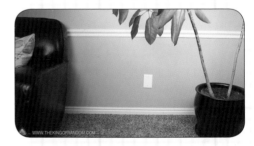

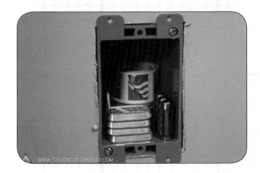

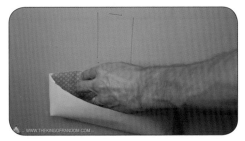

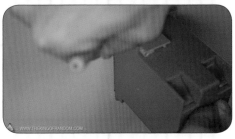

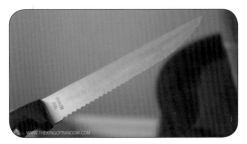

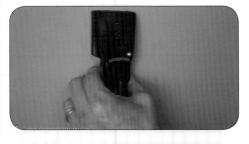

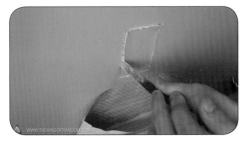

Sometimes the best place to hide something is where people least expect it.

In this project, we're making a super secret safe that only you'll know about.

You'll need one of these extra long electrical gang boxes made for existing walls. You'll also need a blank wall plate, like this.

Step 1: Installation

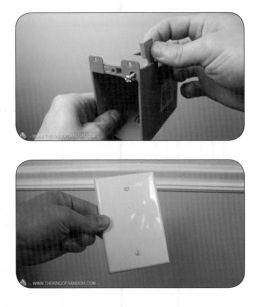

To place the safe, search around your house for a clean section of wall and use a stud finder to locate an area between the studs. When you've found a spot that works, measure a height that matches the outlets nearby and add half an inch.

Next, line up the mark with the bottom left corner of the box and trace around the sides. This is where you'll need to cut into the wall.

I chose to stick an envelope under the markings, so that when cutting into the sheetrock, the envelope catches the dust, reducing the mess that has to be cleaned up later.

It's important to cut carefully and with shallow strokes because there could be electrical wires behind the wall and you don't want to cut them by accident.

Step 2: Securing to the Wall

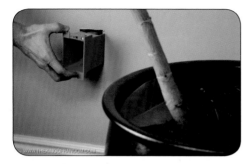

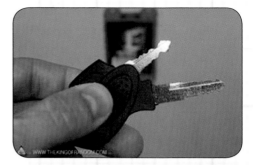

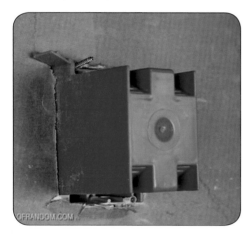

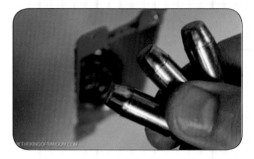

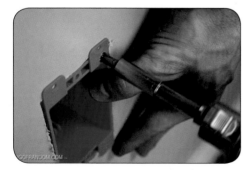

When it's all cut out, you should find that your blue box pushes in perfectly and rests flat against the wall.

When you adjust the screws in the corners, you can see that it tightens the flaps at the back, securing the box tight to the wall.

At this point, you can start loading your safe with something important. Perhaps some stamps you want to save? A set of spare keys? What about emergency ammunition?

Step 3: Hiding Your Treasures

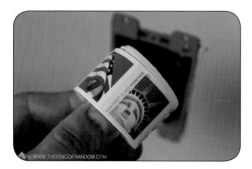

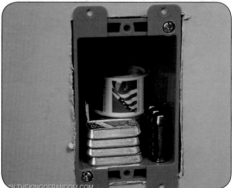

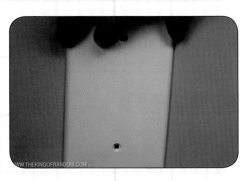

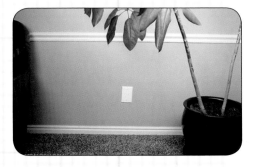

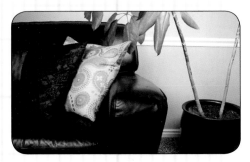

Step 4: Easy Access and Modifications

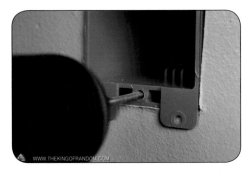

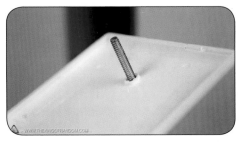

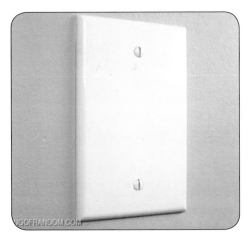

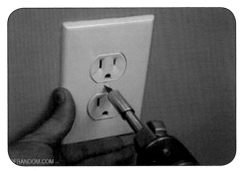

When whatever you put in there is all tucked away, simply add the cover plate and screw it together. Chances are, no one will ever guess there's anything hidden inside.

If you want to go one step further, try pushing some furniture in front of the cover, because out of sight means out of mind.

Now if the time comes where you need to open your safe and you don't have a screwdriver, no problem. Just use the prongs from a plug. The blades fit perfectly into the screw heads, allowing you full and unlimited access.

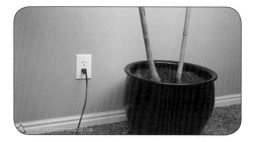

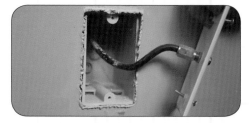

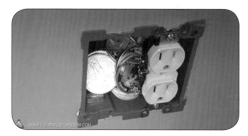

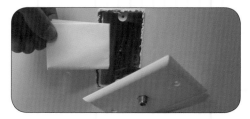

Now there are plenty of modifications you can make to this thing. For example, if you plan on using this a lot and can't be bothered with unscrewing it every time, try drilling out the screw holes with a 9/64" drill bit. Then add a dab of super glue to where the screws meet the cover plate.

This way, the screws will be held fast in place and now you can just line up the holes and press it together in an instant.

If you want this to blend better with the surroundings, try adding an outlet to the front of the box and a finishing plate over that. Now your secret safe looks like all the other outlets in your house.

Have you got so much stuff that you need a bigger safe? Try upgrading to a double-gang. This gives you nearly twice the storage space and installs just as easily as the others.

Step 5: Easy, Free, and Pre-Existing!

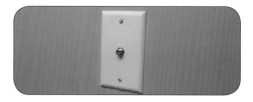

As a final thought, if you don't want to spend the $3 on materials or cut holes in your walls, just look for one of these cable jacks around the house.

The cable's protected, there's plenty of space inside, and it's a great place for hiding things, like your list of computer passwords.

Not only is this option free, but chances are, you've already got them all over the house.

Step 6: Guard Your Secrets

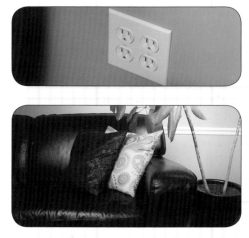

Well, now you know how to make an easy secret safe for hiding important stuff.

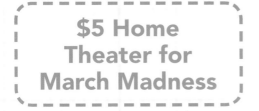

$5 Home Theater for March Madness

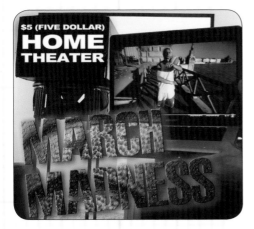

Just in time for March Madness! Here's how to convert your laptop, smartphone, or tablet into a makeshift projector. It's really cheap and can add a bit of creative fun to your next sports party!

This project is geared mainly toward college students looking for a way to turn devices they already have into a projector for sporting events or parties. It's more of a novelty than anything practical, but in my experience, the image is watchable and the idea will hopefully be enjoyed. If anything, it's a party trick you can pull out for your next get-together with friends.

NOTE:

The image projected on the wall will be "mirror image" or "flipped horizontally" from the original image. This will make any text or numbers appear backward. The light from the laptop, smartphone, or tablet is the only source of light, so as the image is made bigger, the intensity of the light on the screen gets weaker until eventually the image becomes indiscernible.

Step 1: What You'll Need

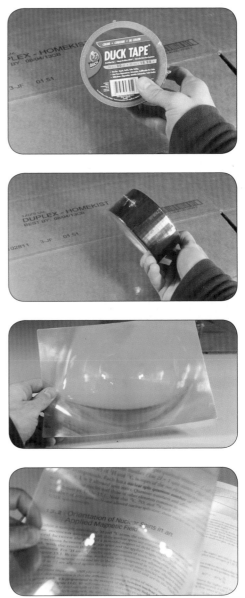

Aside from already owning a laptop, smartphone, or tablet, you're going to need three items to make this projector:
1. Cardboard
2. Duct tape

3. Full-page Fresnel lens

Cardboard: I got my cardboard box at a Walmart. I just went into the photo-lab area and asked if they had any boxes I could use for a project. They had more than they cared to have! I chose one that was a couple feet long, and the front face was just larger than my iPad.

Tape: For tape, I got black duct tape (also from Walmart), but even packing tape or masking tape can work just great!

Fresnel lens: I found my Fresnel lens on eBay for about $3.99. Since then, I've seen them as low as $2.99. The size is somewhere around 8" x 10". These are typically used as full page magnifiers for reading small text.

Step 2: Cutting the Cardboard

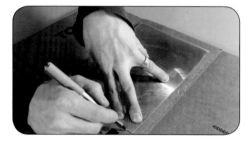

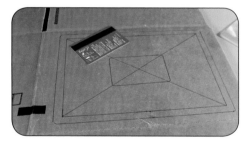

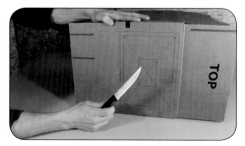

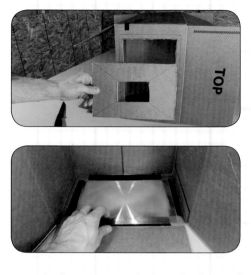

Ideally, we want a hole in the front of the box about ½" smaller than the lens. I used the actual lens as a template to trace around the edges and then drew another rectangle ½" inside the first. It's this inner rectangle that we'll be cutting out, and it should leave a ½" ledge for us to tape the lens onto. You can also use something like a credit card or hotel key to trace a rectangle in the center. When it's all cut out, you should have a left-over piece, as seen in the picture, and you may want to hang onto that.

Now you can use some tape to secure the lens on the inside of the box. **NOTE:**

The grooved part of the lens should be facing inside the box, and the flat smooth side should be facing outward.

Step 3: Finished Projector and Variations for Laptops

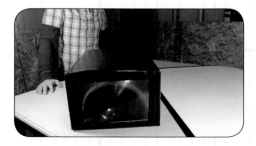

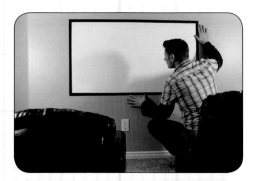

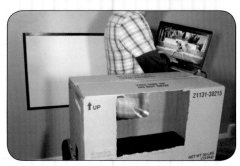

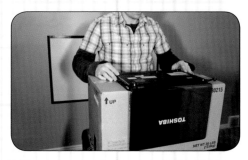

that a hole could be cut on the back of a different box, and the laptop turned upside-down and slid into place. This is by far the quickest and easiest set-up, and the laptop gives the best results because the screen is the biggest and brightest!

Step 4: Get Ready for Your Video!

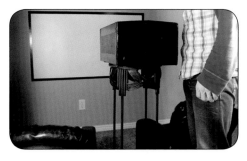

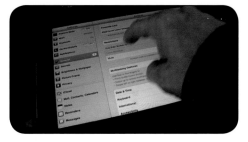

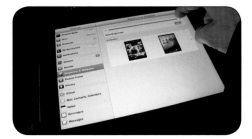

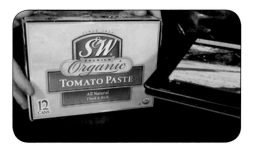

When the lens is set, you can close up the box to give it stability. Your tablet or smartphone will go inside and project outward through the lens.

I gave mine a quick paint job to make it a little nicer, and made a projection screen with a piece of 0.02" Hi-Impact Styrene I got from a sign supply company for just over $2.00. It's 4 feet wide and the black duct tape made a nice border trim on the plastic sheet. I had just enough tape left over to put it up on the wall and rig up a makeshift home theater.

When using a laptop, this configuration will be too small. I found

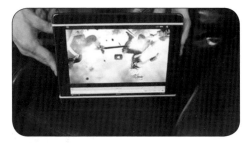

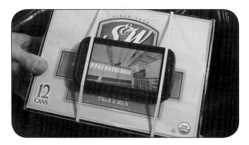

This means that any words or numbers on the screen will still be backward.

Step 5: Success!

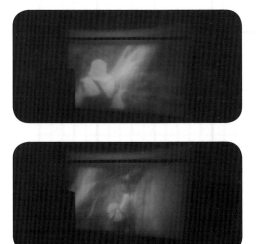

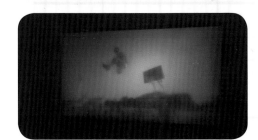

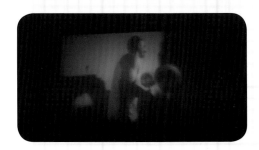

The image that gets projected on the screen will be flipped horizontal and upside-down. You can make it right-side-up by turning your tablet, smartphone or laptop upside down in the projector.

If you're using a tablet like an iPad, you'll also need to go into the settings menu and make sure to lock the rotation of the screen so that it's sideways. Otherwise when you turn it over, the image won't stay upside down.

Whatever device you're using, you'll also need to bring the brightness up to maximum to get the most light. If your phone doesn't have an option to lock the screen, you may need to download an app.

To hold the device in the projector, you'll probably want to find something sturdy, like a couple of text books or a sturdy box. I used a box of tomato paste that was about the size of an iPad.

Using a couple of rubber bands to secure the device in an upside-down position, it's now ready to go in the projector and play your movie!

NOTE:

The image should be right-side-up, but it will still be flipped horizontally.

I found that using a laptop works the best, because the screen is larger to begin with and the brightness level can be turned up. This is good because as the image is made bigger, the intensity of the light on the screen is lessened. An image of 50" is very watchable on a laptop as well as a tablet about the size of an iPad. Of course, the closer you bring the projector to the screen, the smaller the image will be, but the brighter and more focused it will become. I found that if you cover all your windows and close any doors to make sure the room is completely dark, this will help the image appear crisper and brighter.

Because the Fresnel lens is made flat, there are some optical disadvantages that appear in the image. For example, the edges of the screen may be a little blurry while the center is in focus. To address this problem, a shroud can be added to the lens with a rectangular hole in the center about the size of a credit card. This will choke down the aperture and dramatically improve the focus. The trade off is that there will be less light emitted from the projector, so the image on the screen will be dimmed.

A smartphone works the same way, but the screen size can't go much over 20″ or the image is unwatchable. The 15″ worked great and 20″ was ok.

Step 6: Conclusion

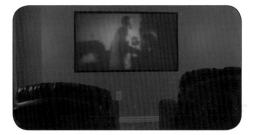

Since the dissipation of the light reduces the brightness on the screen, it's more of a novelty than anything practical, but in my experience, the image is watchable and the idea will hopefully be enjoyed.

If anything, it's a party trick you can pull out for your next get-together with friends.

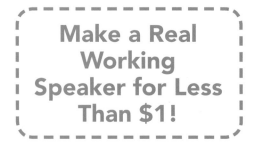

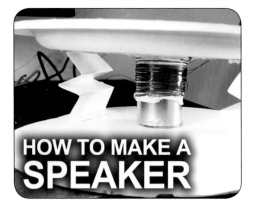

HOW TO MAKE A SPEAKER

Here's how to make a real working paper plate speaker for under a dollar!

$1 Paper Plate Speaker?

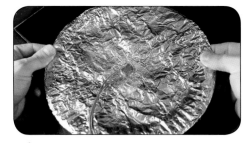

Back in 2007, YouTube user HouseholdHacker posted a parody video on how to make a high-definition speaker for under a buck. MythBusters took on the challenge and busted it.

Although that particular method doesn't seem to work, it doesn't mean you can't make your own speaker for under a dollar. Actually, you can, and it's really easy!

How Does a Speaker Work?

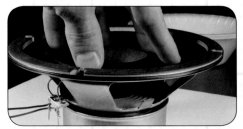

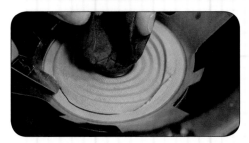

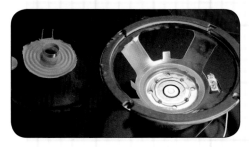

To understand how a speaker works, I took one apart.

In its simplest form, a speaker is just a coil of wire glued to a piece of paper and placed near a permanent magnet. When an alternating current flows through the coiled wire, it is either attracted or repelled by the permanent magnet.

The audio signal from your stereo is a form of alternating current. When attached to a coil of wire and set near a stable magnetic field, the variations in polarity and amplitude will make it vibrate thousands upon thousands of times per second.

If this coiled wire is attached to a diaphragm, the vibrations will push a larger volume of air and generate sound waves that we can hear.

In the pictures above, you can see a paper speaker cone, the yellow spider (which holds the voice coil in place over the magnet), the voice coil with wrappings of magnet wire around it, and a strong permanent magnet at the bottom of the assembly.

The two ends of the voice coil wire are what connect to your stereo system. That's all there is to it! Now let's see if we can make one!

Gather Your Materials

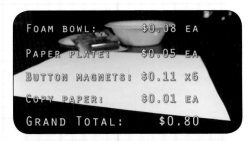

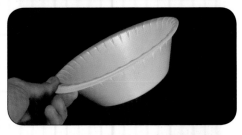

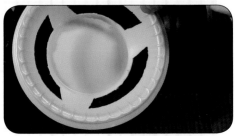

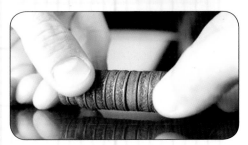

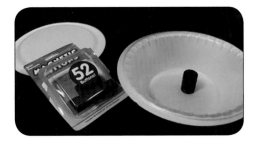

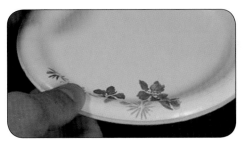

For this project, let's use:
- A foam bowl for the speaker basket
- A paper plate that fits onto the top of the bowl as the speaker cone
- Button magnets that can be stacked into a cylinder
- A sheet of printer paper to form the voice coil support
- Magnet wire to form the actual voice coil (Magnet wire is thin enameled copper wire and can be salvaged from many electronic devices for free, or bought at places like Radio Shack)
- A hot glue gun and some scissors.

Just for fun, I used a knife and cut holes in the sides of the foam bowl so it looked more like a speaker cone.

NOTE:

None of these materials are sold individually because they only come in packs, but if the pieces are pro-rated, the cost is around eighty cents per speaker!

I found some magnet wire inside an old TV. Many of the small transformers on the circuit board were loaded with the perfect wire for this

WARNING:

Be aware if you are salvaging electronics at home. Capacitors on the circuit boards may still hold a charge and pose a risk of electric shock. This project should not be attempted without adult supervision and adequate training.

Make an Eighty-Cent Speaker!

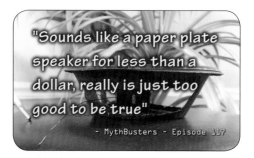

"Sounds like a paper plate speaker for less than a dollar, really is just too good to be true"
- MythBusters - Episode 117

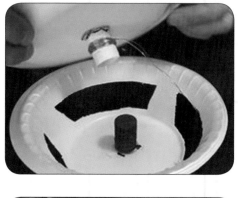

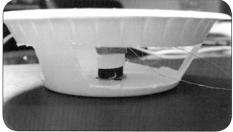

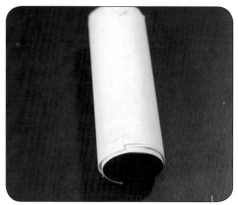

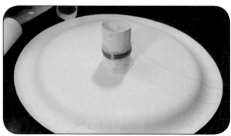

You get what you pay for, but it works!

Step 1: Stack about five to six button magnets to form a one-inch to two-inch cylinder

Step 2: Cut a strip of paper and roll it around the stack of magnets, and then tape it to itself.

Step 3: Cut a second strip of paper and roll it over the first, and then tape it to itself.

NOTE:

The two pieces of paper should not be connected to each other. Instead, they should be able to slide apart freely. The inner paper is going to serve as a spacer, because when it's removed, it will create a slight gap between the top tube and the magnets.

Step 4: Wrap about 50 turns of wire around the tube. It doesn't have to be super tight, but should be firm.

Step 5: Secure the wire coil in place with some hot glue.

Step 6: Pull the stack of magnets and inner coil of paper out of the tube.

You should now have a hollow tube with a winding of wire around it. This is your "voice coil."

Step 7: Glue the voice coil to the bottom side of a paper plate.

Step 8: Cut the voice coil to a length that will slide over the magnet stack, and hover the wire coil near the top of the magnets.

Step 9: Fit the paper plate with the voice coil over the top of the magnets and glue the plate in place.

I chose to paint the speaker black in an attempt to make it look a little better.

Step 10: Remove the coating from the tips of the wires. You can use sandpaper or an open flame to burn off the enamel.

Step 11: Hook your speaker up to a stereo with a built-in amplifier and press play.

You should hear your music playing out of your paper plate! It's not going to be very loud because any magnet you can get for this cheap is going to be very poor quality. But it does work and it's a fun project!

Troubleshooting:

If you don't hear anything, double check your connections. The two wires from the voice coil should connect to the positive and negative terminals of one channel of your system. It doesn't really matter which wire goes where, as both will work.

Your stereo will also need to have a built-in audio amplifier to push a higher wattage to the plate. If you're trying to run this from your iPhone or MP3 player, you might hear a faint noise, but your results will be much better if you first amplify the power output.

If you still don't hear anything, your wire is damaged (shorting out or broken), you don't have a good connection with your wires to your audio source, or your magnets aren't strong enough.

What difference would a stronger magnet make? Let's find out.

What Makes the Speaker Better?

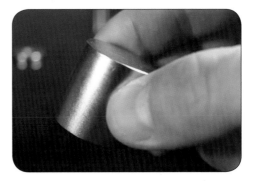

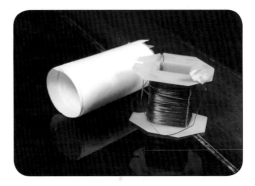

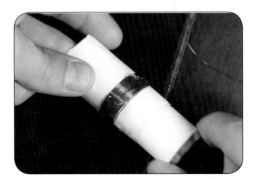

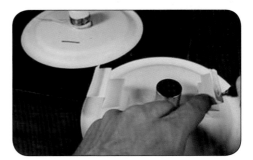

make a real working speaker for less than $1!

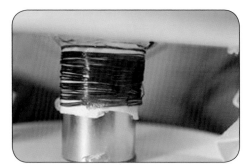

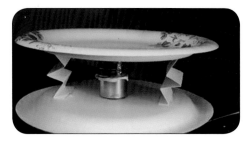

The strength of your magnet plays a huge part on the strength of the sound.

I made another speaker using a Neodymium magnet. These are among the world's strongest magnets.

The voice coil is made the same way by wrapping paper and wire around the magnet, and then removing the voice coil shell and cutting it to size.

I used scrap wire I found on an old sump-pump motor for this one.

This time, instead of using a foam bowl for the speaker basket, I just glued the magnet to another paper plate for a base, and made some accordion-style supports to hold the coil over the magnet.

When the leads were connected and the music turned up, I was amazed at the results! It was rocking out!

Pouring water into the plate shows just how powerful the vibrations are with the stronger magnetic field. It also makes quite a mess.

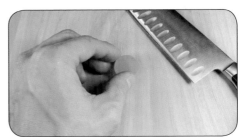

How to Make a One-Way Check Valve for Cheap!

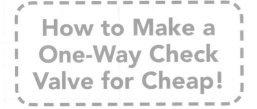

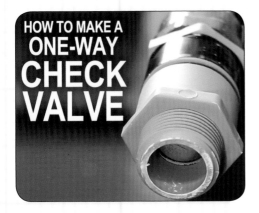

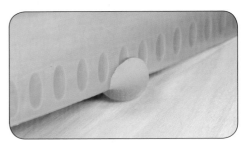

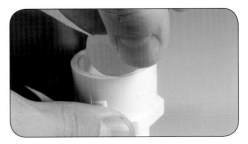

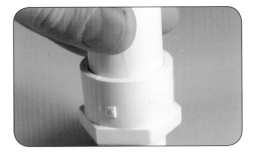

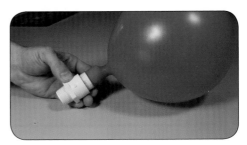

It's summer. If you're going to build yourself a water-gun or a water pump, you'll need some check valves. These should work for you PVC building enthusiasts!

The most expensive parts of a water pump or DIY Super Soaker are usually the check valves. In this project, we're making some from scratch for as little as thirty-five cents each.

WARNING:

The pressure tests and claims made on these check-valves are based solely on my personal experiences. Individual results may vary, and caution and care should be taken when loading the valves with high pressure. The risk of higher pressures is that the balls may be forced from the adaptor, shooting out like projectiles. High pressures may also cause the ball to lock up, preventing normal operation of the valve or possibly even structural failure of the valve altogether. These valves are not made to be used in any heavy duty operations. Use of this content is at your own risk.

how to make a one-way check valve for cheap!

In this project, I'll show two different ways to make a simple check valve. One is easy (simple but for low-pressure applications only), and one a little more complex (good up to around 50–60 PSI).

In both cases, the valves will share two common parts.

1. One ¾" male PVC slip adaptor.
2. A length of ¾" PVC tubing (1½" or longer).

To make the quick and easy valve:

1. Find a ¾" rubber bouncy ball and slowly cut off the top one third.
2. Place the ball inside the PVC slip adaptor with the round side facing down, and the flat side facing up.
3. Press the ¾" PVC tube into the slip adaptor down far enough that it is firm and tight, but leaving enough room for the ball to move around a bit inside.

That's it!

For low-pressure applications, like blowing up balloons, this little device will make your little kids feel like balloon-blowing champions.

The valve allows air into the balloon, and when you stop blowing, the valve closes and the air stays in the balloon indefinitely.

A Little More Complex

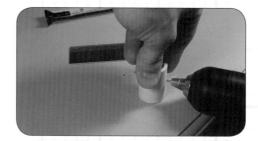

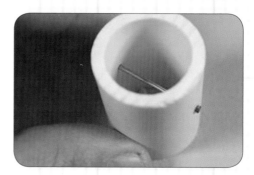

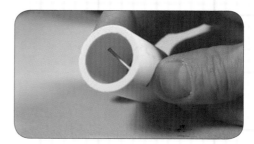

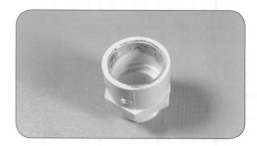

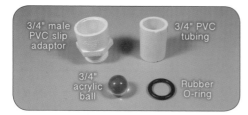

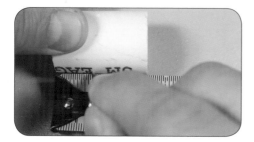

For this valve, we'll use the harder plastic ball and an O ring. These are made to be a little more durable.

Prepare the tube:

1. Start by taking a piece of ¾" PVC tubing (minimum 1½") and measure ⅝" from the bottom.
2. Drill a hole at the mark that goes through both walls of the tubing.

3. Find a strong piece of metal, like a thick paperclip or a nail to insert into the holes.
4. Trim the head off the nail so that both ends of the nail or paperclip are flush with the outside walls of the tube.

NOTE:

This valve can be built into any length of PVC pipe you choose.

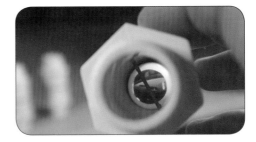

Prepare the slip adaptor for connecting, and then:

1. Prime the inside walls of the adaptor, as well as the part of the tube that will slide into it.
2. Insert the O ring and plastic ball into the adaptor and check for a good fit and good seal.
3. Glue the parts that were primed, and slide the tube into the adaptor until the nail holes dip just below the surface.

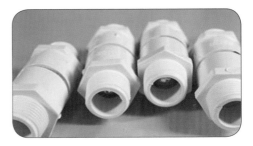

NOTE:

Don't press so hard that the ball is trapped in the closed position. You will need a little gap for the ball so the valve can open and close.

4. Let the cement cure for about two hours before use.

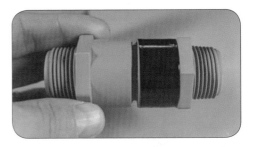

Make Them Multi-Use

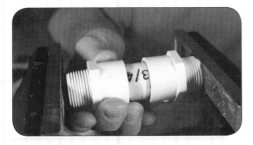

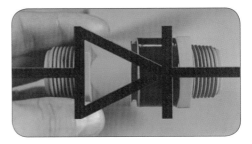

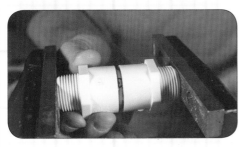

To make these valves more convenient, I tried adding another slip adaptor to the other end of the 1½" pipe. This increases the cost by thirty-four cents, but it's worth it.

I chose 1½" as the pipe length because when the adaptors are pushed together, it leaves only a very small gap and makes the unit very compact. In the picture, you can see the ball held in the unit by the adaptor and the retaining nail preventing it from rolling it out of the tube.

I also gave them a quick paint job with some spray paint and added electrical tape to one side so the direction of flow can be easily identified, similar to the schematic symbol for an electrical diode.

Testing and Applications

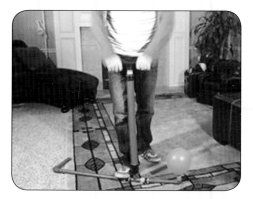

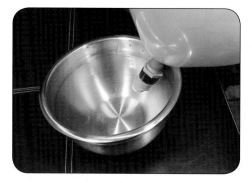

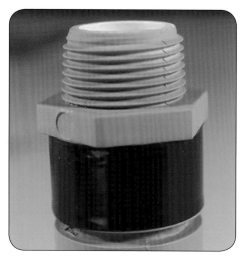

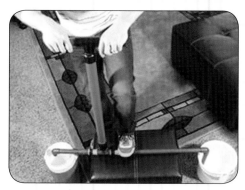

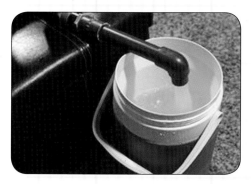

To test your valve, use it to blow up a balloon. The balloon should stay inflated even when you stop blowing.

Place the valve into a bowl of water. If there is any air escaping at all, you will see little bubbles coming from the valve. If there are no air bubbles, that means your valve is both air-tight and water-tight.

Because we used the slip adaptors, the ends of the connections are threaded and allow the valves to be integrated

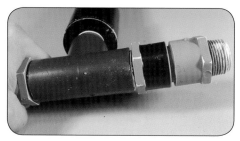

into any system and switched around at will.

My motivation in building these valves stemmed from a desire to build a PVC water pump, but the check valves were around ten dollars each. That seemed a little steep for a PVC build, so while looking for alternative options, I settled on this design, which is about the cheapest, while still being practical and useful.

I tried using two of these check valves to make a PVC water pump. It can be used as an air pump, a vacuum pump, or a water pump that will pump up to five gallons per minute.

In my testing, the valves work great with air and water. Air pressures up to 60 PSI seemed to be fine for normal operation, while pressures above 60 PSI occasionally caused the ball to lock into the O Ring, and required substantial "back pressure" to unlock it.

In Closing

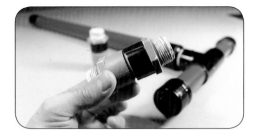

If you try using rubber bouncy balls as the valve mechanism, only use them in very low-pressure applications, like blowing up balloons, and possibly for improvised water guns. Relatively high-pressure used with these balls seems to eventually force them out of the adaptor and can shoot them out at surprising velocities.

Overall, I'm really happy with the valves because they can be fit into any part of a PVC system, and can be duplicated quickly, easily, and for very, very low cost.

Section 5

Water, Ice, and Dry Ice Hacks

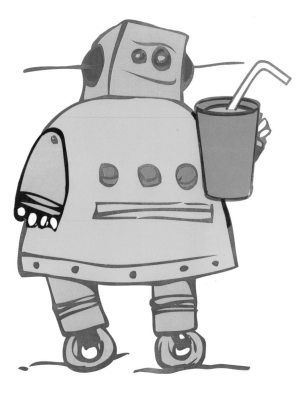

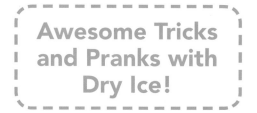
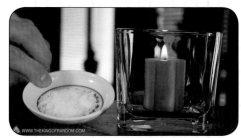

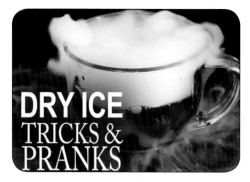

DRY ICE TRICKS & PRANKS

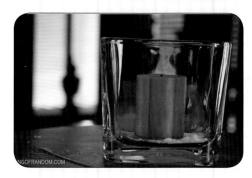

You don't have to wait for Halloween to play with dry ice. Here are five "non-Halloween" ways to use dry ice for tricks and pranks.

Where in the world do you get dry ice? Try searching DryIceDirectory.com for a location near you.

WARNING:

Use content at your own risk. Dry ice is −78°C and is very cold and poses risk for instant frostbite on bare skin. To avoid frostbite on bare skin, handling of dry ice should be approached with caution and attempted with gloves or other protection. There are risks associated with these projects that require adult supervision.

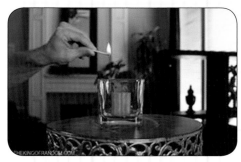

Impossible Candle Relight

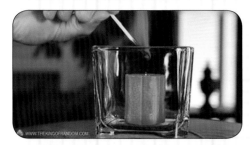

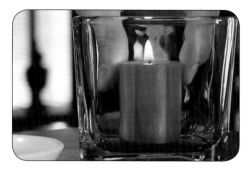

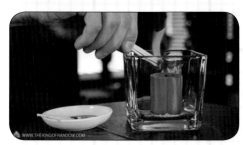

For this prank, take a flaming candle and place it down into a container like a bowl or a glass.

Carefully pour some crushed dry ice down around the base of the candle. And within just a few seconds, you'll notice the flame goes out and the gas turns completely invisible.

Now challenge one of your friends to try and relight the candle inside the glass. They won't be able to do it and they'll have no idea why. Even after multiple attempts, the flame goes out every time.

Now simply blow into the top of the glass to push the gas out and show your friends that it really isn't that difficult after all. The candle will relight easily.

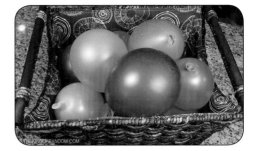

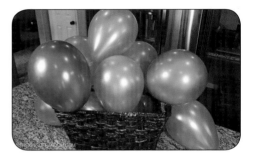

Self-Inflating Party Balloons

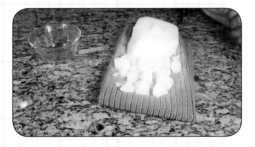

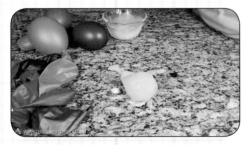

For this trick, find a block of dry ice and break it into pieces the size of small rocks.

Carefully place one or two of the pieces inside of a balloon and tie it off. You'll notice the balloon begins to inflate all by itself.

Now try doing this with a bunch of other balloons and throw them all into a basket.

Over the course of about twenty-five minutes, the balloons will keep growing until you've got a basket overflowing.

Ziploc Poppers

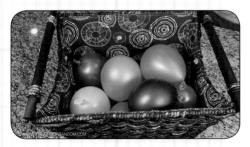

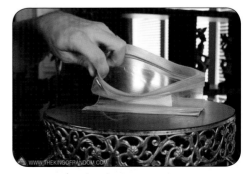

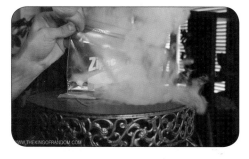

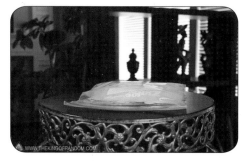

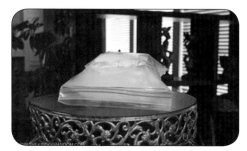

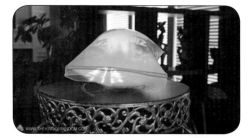

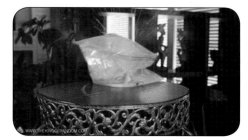

Start this prank by opening up a Ziploc bag and adding a few chunks of dry ice followed by a little bit of warm water.

Now seal the bag so it's completely air-tight, and find a place to hide it. After a minute or two, the bag will be completely pressurized and ready to explode. It will make an impressive bang! Who could you scare with this?

Now this is completely safe, and you can do it with heavy duty freezer bags as well. The plastic is a little thicker, so a bit more pressure can build before they go off.

Squealing Spoons and Shivering Quarters

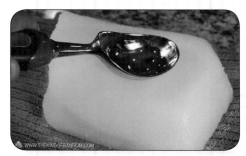

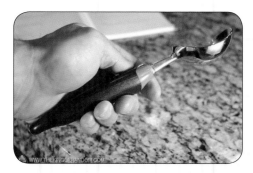

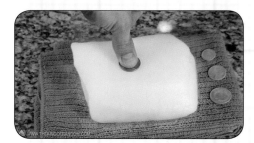

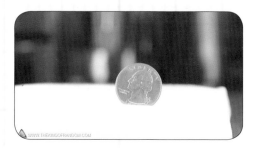

Levitating Bubbles

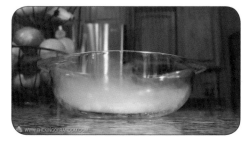

For this party trick, take a large metal spoon and press it down into a block of dry ice. It lets out an awful squeal and people will beg you to stop. You can make a quarter scream the same way. Just lay it flat on the ice, and press down into it. By the way, it's probably a good idea to use gloves, because these get very cold very quickly.

For a bonus trick, try sticking the quarter in sideways. It'll start shaking uncontrollably.

For this last trick, add some crushed dry ice into a large clear bowl. Now wait for the gas to fill it up and turn invisible.

At this point, try blowing the biggest bubble you can, and drop it right in the center.

Instead of popping on the bottom, it levitates around in mid-air, and will make your friends wonder, "What kind of sorcery is this?"

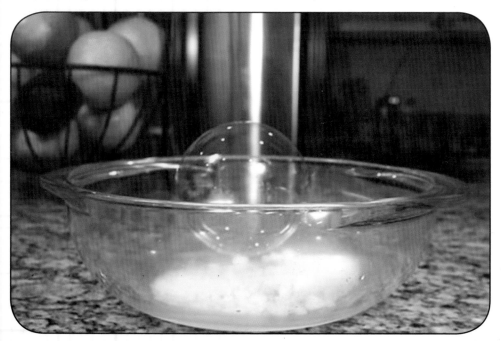

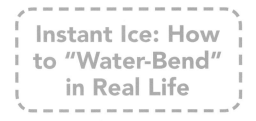

Instant Ice: How to "Water-Bend" in Real Life

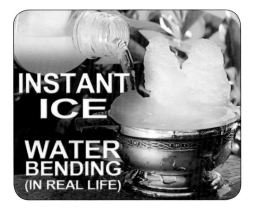

Pour a glass of water and watch it turn to ice instantly! This step-by-step tutorial will show you everything you need to know about instant ice. This is how to "water-bend" in real life!

"Super Cool" Water Trick

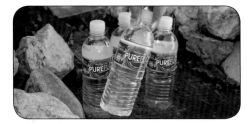

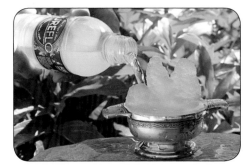

A couple of years ago, a friend at work told me he left water bottles outside overnight in freezing temperatures. Then he got the water to freeze instantly by shaking them.

I was fascinated by the idea, and began to research the online resources demonstrating the effect of super-cooled water, and began to experiment with it on my own. I can confirm, along with hundreds of others, that this phenomenon is legit, and here's how to do it step-by-step!

1. Find some purified water (the easiest place to find this is an unopened bottle of water).
2. Put it in the freezer for the exact amount of time to super-cool it (more on this later).
3. Initiate nucleation of the ice crystals (easier than it sounds).

How to Super-Cool Water

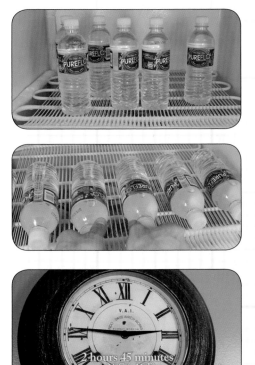

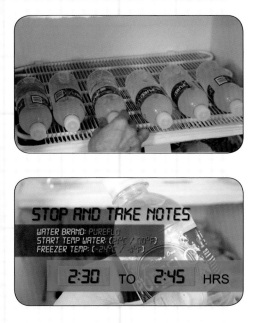

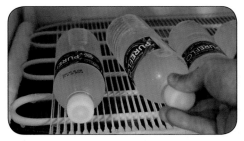

all the bottles worked consistently from between two and a half hours and two hours and forty-five minutes.

How to Test Your Super-Cooled Water

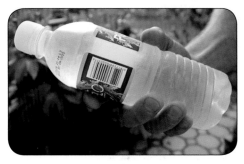

Every bottle is going to be a little bit different. Some factors that affect the time to freeze are:

- Volume of water in the bottle.
- Size and shape of the bottle.
- Temperature of water before it goes in the freezer.
- Temperature of the freezer.
- Position of the bottle in the freezer.
- Impurities in the water.

The easiest way to find out the ideal freeze time for your bottles is to start with bottles at room temperature and put multiple bottles in the freezer at the same time. This will increase your chances for success.

To determine the formula for your specific bottles:

- Make a note of the time.
- Check your bottles after ninety minutes, and thereafter every fifteen minutes until one freezes.
- Mark the time of the frozen bottle and subtract fifteen minutes.

Your specific bottles should work within this window of opportunity. In my case, the first bottle froze after two hours and forty-five minutes, and I found

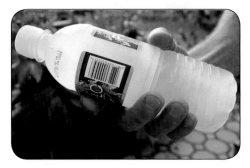

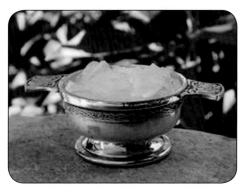

In Another Container

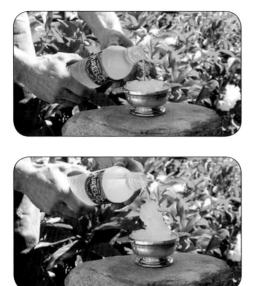

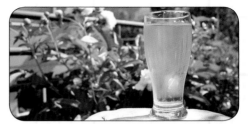

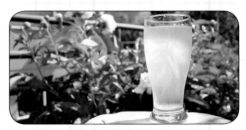

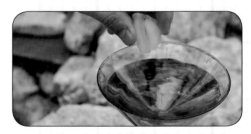

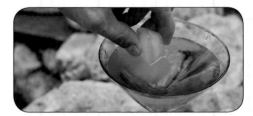

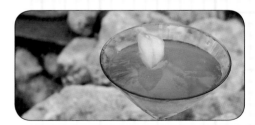

The rest of the unfrozen bottles in the freezer should be super-cooled and ready for action.

When you take them from the freezer, be very gentle. They are super sensitive and can freeze with even the slightest jolt. To test one, just give it a whack on the bottle anywhere you want. If you hit it hard enough, you should see the water instantly begin to freeze from the top to the bottom. The result will be a clear liquid turning to an opaque white, as seen in the pictures.

You can also freeze the water using a piece of ice as a nucleation point. Just pour the water on top of the ice and watch your ice pillars grow right before your eyes! If they don't grow very fast, try leaving your bottles in the freezer for another ten minutes. If your bottles are freezing with only a slight touch or before you want them to, try taking your bottles out of the freezer five minutes earlier.

As the water freezes, it actually releases latent heat into the ice and the temperature warms up to just below freezing. This leaves you with a delicious edible slush with the consistency of a wet snowball.

You can try pouring your water into an extremely clean glass. If it's still liquid at this point, try dropping an ice cube into the center and watch the whole thing crystallize. You can do the same thing by just holding an ice cube on the surface of the water.

Colored Ice

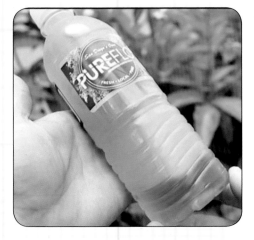

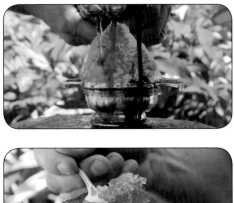

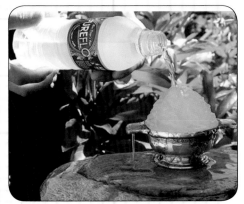

I found you could color your crystallization by adding a couple of drops of food coloring to the water before they go in the freezer. In this case, I used two drops of blue food coloring.

I tried pouring out an entire bottle on a bed of ice to form an "instant snow cone," and then used some juice from melted freeze pops as makeshift syrup—a fun and entertaining treat for a hot summer day!

Well, there you have it! That's how to freeze water instantly like a "water-bending" master.

How to Make Dry Ice with a Fire Extinguisher!

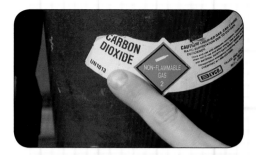

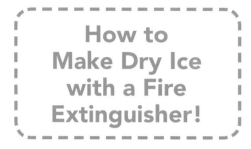

Here's how to make dry ice at home or wherever you feel like it! All you need is a pillow case and a CO2 fire extinguisher.

This project was inspired by: Theo Gray (Mad Science)

WARNING:

Dry ice is extremely cold (–78°C/–109°F) and can cause instant frostbite to exposed skin. This project should not be attempted without adult supervision and adequate training. Misuse or careless use of tools or projects may result in serious injury. Use of this content is at your own risk.

Getting the Equipment

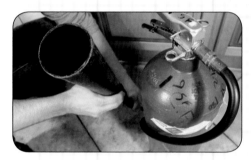

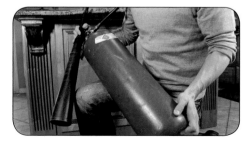

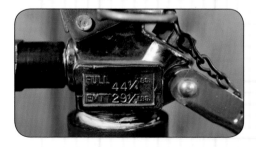

To make dry ice, you need to secure a ready source of compressed liquid CO2. How about a CO2 fire extinguisher?

Some fire extinguishers utilize CO2 as the medium for suppressing fires because it's very clean and doesn't leave behind any residue. When pressurized liquid CO2 is quickly depressurized,

108

the CO2 expands to a gas and cools its surroundings. This is called adiabatic cooling. Because the CO2 sublimates directly into a gas, there's no mess to clean up after discharge!

Where to find one:

I called around to some fire equipment companies asking about CO2 fire extinguishers. I hadn't seen these types of extinguishers much and was looking for where I could buy one used or rent one just for experimenting.

By chance, one man I talked to said he had a 15-pound CO2 extinguisher in storage, which he would give to me for free! If you don't get as lucky, try calling a company that recharges CO2 extinguishers and ask them if you can rent one or borrow one for a science project.

Most fire extinguishers you see are filled with dry chemical. These are NOT what you want. It has to be carbon dioxide. You can distinguish a CO2 fire extinguisher in a few different ways:

- Look for stickers or markings on the side of the tank that indicate "carbon dioxide" or "CO2."
- Look for a servicing sticker or tag with a hole punched next to "CO2."
- Look for an unusually large discharge horn. This is an oversized large black nozzle at the end of the hose.
- Not having pressure gauges is also a good indication.

These types of extinguishers aren't typically in public view. They are mainly found in restaurant kitchens, mechanical rooms, and in areas that hold sensitive equipment like computers. Interestingly enough, the CO2 is "food-grade CO2."

Carbon dioxide fire extinguishers are usually referred to in terms of pounds. For example, a 15-pound CO2 extinguisher is charged with a 15-pound weight of liquid CO2, and this can be identified by markings on the handle showing the full and empty weights.

Making Dry Ice

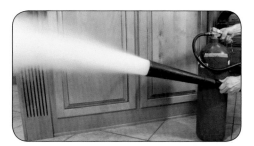

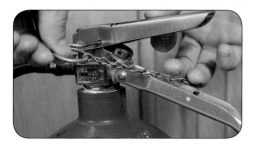

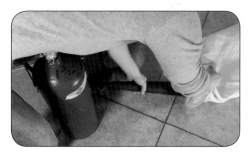

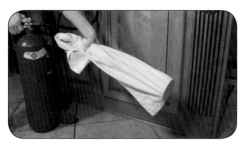

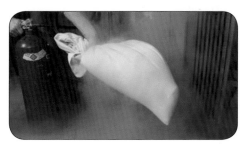

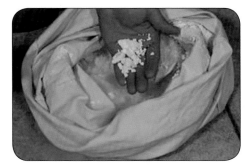

Operation of the fire extinguisher is the same as any other. Just remove the locking pin and press down on the handle.

What you'll see is a forceful jet of carbon dioxide vapor blasting from the discharge horn. The gas is extremely cold and may take your breath away if you get too close.

The trick to getting dry ice:

Here's the trick—trap the cold!

Using a porous cloth material, like a pillowcase, cover the end of the discharge horn and pull up all the loose material.

When you have a good grip, give it a four- to six-second blast! Hang on tight, because there will be a lot of pressure pumping into your pillowcase and you need to keep it from blowing away.

Oh yeah, it's also going to be pretty loud, so warn your family before you do it. That's speaking from experience!

When you remove the pillowcase, there will be a solid buildup at the bottom of the bag, as well as on the nozzle. Make sure to save that into the bag, and then open it up to see what you got!

I found chunks of dry ice snow, and digging down near the bottom, I found enough to make a good sized dry ice snowball!

Dry ice is –78°C, so using insulated gloves is recommended. I didn't use gloves, and while I did feel a little cold nip every now and again, I found for the most part that if I kept the ice moving

around quickly, it didn't have a chance to sit long enough to give me frostbite.

The dry ice sublimates directly from a solid to a gas, so in an attempt to make it last longer, I transferred it to a small bowl to keep it together and reduce the exposed surface area.

Things to Do with Dry Ice!

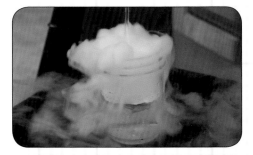

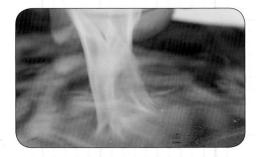

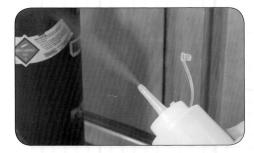

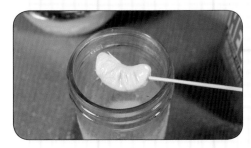

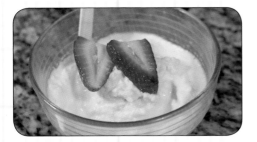

I tried making a poor man's version of liquid nitrogen, which actually flash-froze an orange!

The remainder of the dry ice went into making a nice batch of carbonated ice cream. Delicious!

Other Projects

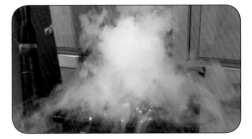

The classic dry-ice experiment is to place a few chunks in a container and pour some warm water over it.

This creates a flowing fog effect that is common at Halloween parties in something like a witches brew. The fog can even be poured out to form a cascading waterfall of mist that will flow gracefully over your countertop. The best part is that there's no mess to clean up!

I put a few chunks in a condiment container and screwed on a lid with a vent hole in the cap. When I shook it up, the reaction accelerated and I got a little CO_2 geyser rocketing out of the top! The pressure was enough to make me wonder if it could be used to drive a small motor of some sort?

Well, there's how to make "on-demand" dry ice in a portable and "do-it-yourself" fashion.

Saying that, I should mention that it cost just under thirty dollars to refill the tank to get about five pounds of dry ice. Contrasting that with the cost of dry ice at the local grocery store ($1/lb.) doesn't make financial sense, but this method is much more fun!

How to Convert Water into Fuel by Building a DIY Oxyhydrogen Generator

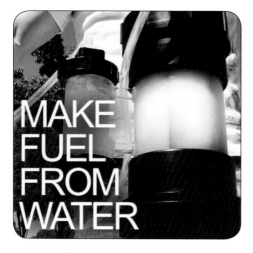

Here's how to build a sexy-looking generator that uses electricity to convert water into an extremely powerful fuel! In this project, you'll learn how to build an OxyHydrogen generator from scratch.

What Is an OxyHydrogen Generator?

An oxyhydrogen generator, like this one, uses electricity from your car battery to split water into hydrogen and oxygen gases (electricity + $2H2O$ —> $2H2 + O2$). Together, these make a fuel that is much more powerful than gasoline, and the only emission released is water!

Of course, to be a completely clean fuel, the electricity used to generate the gas needs to be from a clean source. Solar, wind, or water power could be a few examples.

NOTE:

The amount of electrical energy required to make the gas is more than the energy you can obtain from it. This is NOT an energy generator so much as it is an energy converter.

Getting Metal for the Generator Plates

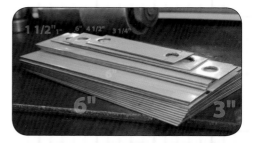

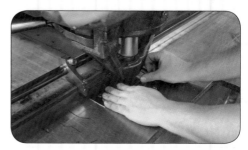

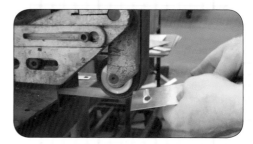

For this project, you're going to need some stainless steel and some ABS pipe fittings. I visited a local fabrication company, and not only did they have plenty of scrap metal to choose from, they were even willing to help me cut it to custom sizes. A job that would have taken me hours with a pair of tin snips and a hacksaw took only a matter of minutes with their equipment.

I used 20-gauge stainless steel, and with the help of their hydraulic punch, cut precise holes in the tops and bottoms of the plates. When finished, I had twelve plates measuring 3" x 6", four plates at 1½" x 6", and three 1" connector bands that were 6", 4½" and 3¼". A belt sander was used for smoothing down the jagged edges around the hole.

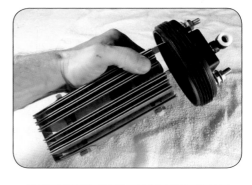

Increasing the Plates' Surface Area

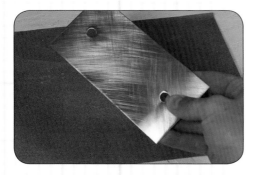

Next, I used 100-grit sandpaper to sand each of the plates diagonally. You can see the "X" pattern I sanded into both sides of the plates. This increases the surface area of the plate and will assist in producing more gas.

Configuring the Plate Assembly

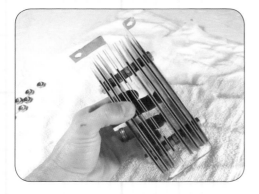

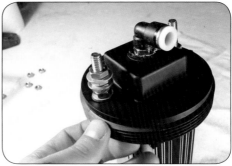

The plates are joined in a configuration so that the two inner plates are connected to one electrical terminal, and the two outer plates connected to the other terminal. Plastic rods, plastic washers, and stainless steel nuts help to form the proper electrical connections.

The generator plates are assembled in the order of plate, plastic washers, plate, stainless steel jam nuts until eight plates have been connected.

When the plates are assembled, a 4" ABS cleanout plug is attached at the top with some stainless steel bolts.

Making the Generator Body

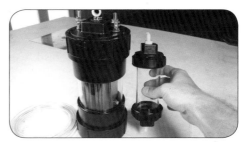

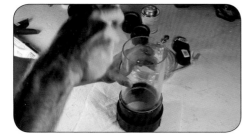

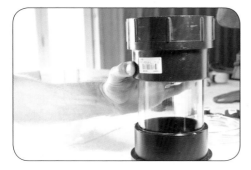

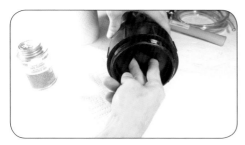

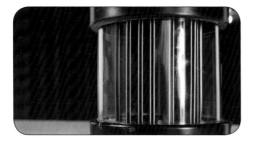

Making Clips for the Bubbler

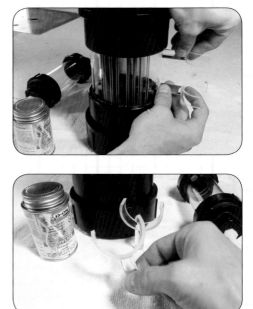

Clips can be made from scrap acrylic or ABS tubing and glued to the side of the body.

To make these clips, I cut ¾" off the 2" tubing I used to make the bubbler, and then cut the top ⅓" off to form a claw. These were then cemented to acrylic rods, and attached to the side of the generator body.

Adding a Check Valve

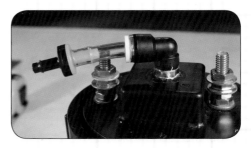

The body is made from two 4" ABS cleanout adapters with a 4" plug inverted and cemented into the bottom. A 4" tube of acrylic or ABS makes the body, and the generator plates and cap screw down into the top.

A water bubbler is made in a similar fashion out of 2" clear acrylic tubing, but needs a way to clip onto the side.

Some poly tube and a one-way check valve is added to the top elbow, making sure the valve will let gas out, but nothing back in.

Making the Electrolyte

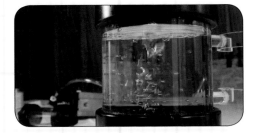

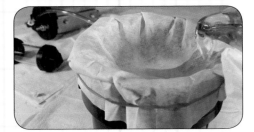

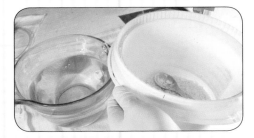

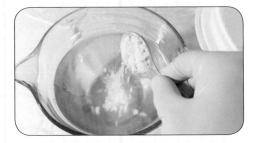

NOTE:

Potassium Hydroxide is caustic and can burn the skin. Avoid direct contact!

Finishing Touches

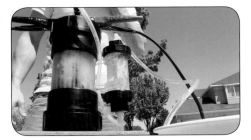

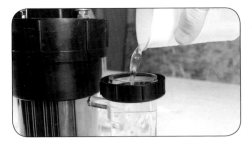

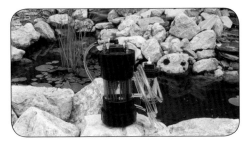

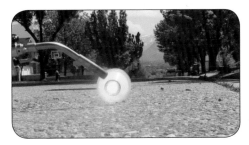

The electrolyte is distilled water and about two to four teaspoons of KOH (potassium hydroxide). Salt or baking soda could also be used but may dirty and corrode the plates over time.

I stirred the KOH flakes into the water, and then used a coffee filter to strain the solution into the generator casing (after it had been cleaned thoroughly).

Water is added to the bubbler, then the cap is put back on and the poly tubes are hooked up.

I tested it out with a 12-volt car battery and some jumper cables. The gas formed is collected in a small water bottle and ignited with a flame.

On 12 volts, this produces about 1.5 LPM. I also hooked it to two car batteries in series, and on this higher 24 voltage, the system produced over 5 LPM and filled up a gallon milk jug in 38 seconds!

NOTE:

Higher voltages allow more current to flow through the system, and it heats up quickly over time. If allowed to continue, there is a risk the plastic casing will melt from prolonged exposure to high temperatures.

How Powerful Is the Gas?

This system was not designed for use in a vehicle, but more as a device to demonstrate the electrolysis of water and what the gas can do.

Section 6

Energizing Hacks

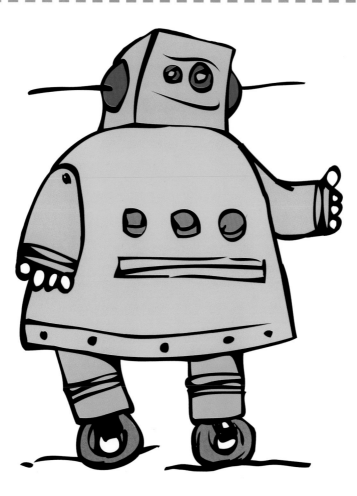

┌──────────────────────────┐
│ **The Scariac**   │
│ **(Poor Man's**   │
│ **Variable Power**   │
│ **Controller)**   │
└──────────────────────────┘

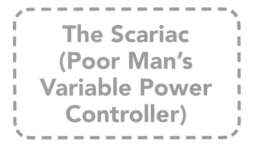

Variac versus Scariac

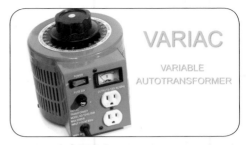

VARIAC

VARIABLE
AUTOTRANSFORMER

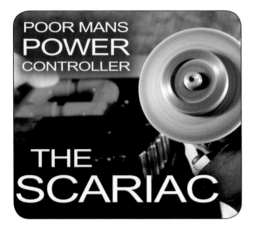

POOR MANS
POWER
CONTROLLER

THE
SCARIAC

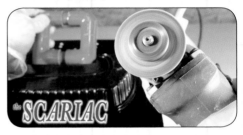

Mixing water with electricity is risky and can be lethal. However, in this project we're using it to make one of the cheapest kinds of power controller. The Scariac.

WARNING:

This project is extremely dangerous and should only be attempted by those highly skilled in working with electricity. High voltages and high currents passing through the water provide an open hazard of electrocution and may cause death. This design does not include any electrical ground. This system is not recommended as a safe device. Its purpose, rather, is to regulate electrical current in a simple and low-cost way. Toxic gases may be released from the solution during operation. This project should not be attempted without adult supervision and adequate training. Misuse or careless use of tools or projects may result in serious injury. Use at your own risk.

I needed a way to adjust the power running to my homemade stick welding system. Even with enough power to the welder, the main problem was finding a system that could vary electrical current without costing an arm and a leg.

In a tight situation, it's good to be aware of options, and that's why I was happy to learn about the idea of the water resistor.

The idea is to use a water-based medium as an electrolytic resistor. A bit of electrolyte is added to the solution to make it slightly conductive, and when two electrodes are placed in the solution, they allow more or less current to flow, depending on whether there are closer or farther apart.

"How-I-Did" Versus "How-to"

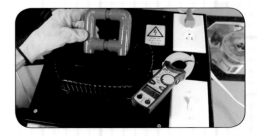

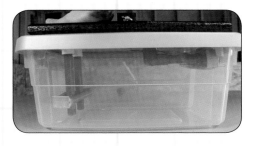

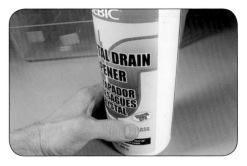

In its simplest form, this device is just a glorified version of two wires in a bucket of water.

Although I've taken thought to minimize risks in operation, I have to stress that I don't consider this device safe or foolproof. It has the potential to be lethal, and even though I show step-by-step how it was made, this is more of a "how-I-did" project rather than a "how-to."

The system has a power lever to vary current output, and a loop of wire for connecting an ammeter. The outlet on the board is where the devices plug in, and the switch acts as a kill-switch to turn the device completely on or off at will.

ADDITIONAL WARNING:

There is no grounding wire connected, and always possibility of failure in any part of the system, so extreme caution and respect is needed when operating. The device doesn't have any internal fuse/circuit breaker/current limiting device so there is also risk of fire if the system shorted out and your home circuit protection system fails. This fire could potentially happen inside the walls of your home.

Electrolyte as Variable Resistor

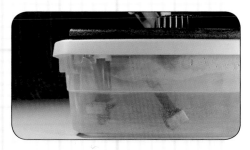

I used a water-based medium for the variable resistance, two gallons of tap water (distilled water will also work great, but is more expensive), and ¼ teaspoon of 100 percent lye (NaOH). Even though the amount of lye is very low, it makes the water conduct very quickly. I found my lye in a drain cleaner from the hardware store—100 percent lye, in fact!

Any salt could probably be used as an electrolyte, but using something like table salt (NaCl) seemed to introduce the possibility of generating Chlorine gas, and that's why I went with the NaOH instead.

Additional Considerations

During operation, the electrolysis does produce some gas. However, it seems to be minimal when supplying with AC power. DC would be a much greater concern.

The system is also open (ventilated), so any gas generation escapes quickly. In my experience, this doesn't give hydrogen and oxygen gases enough time to build up to a dangerous level, and I wasn't able to achieve any gas explosions, even at ultra high power settings, despite trying. However, it is good to be aware of the risks and operate in a well-ventilated area as a precaution.

Well, there you have it! That's how I sacrificed safety to build a variable power controller on a very small budget.

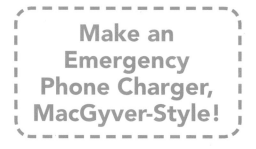

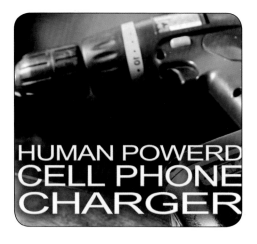

In this video, you'll learn how to "MacGyver" a 40-watt electrical generator from a cordless drill and a few household items. Here's how to charge a phone, illuminate small lights, and make electricity in a pinch.

NOTE:

This project is intended to be a "bare bones" approach to generating electricity in a tight situation. There are no voltage regulators, no diodes, and no capacitors to smooth the current. There may be a risk of overheating and damaging equipment when operating electrical devices without a proper circuit recommended by the manufacturer.

It worked fine for me, but if you try this on your phone, make sure you understand and are comfortable with the risks. Back up your data in case your phone is adversely affected and your data or equipment is damaged as a result.

Household Items

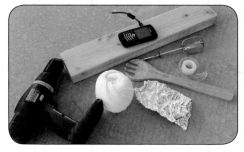

There's no charge for this electricity! All you'll need for this project is a cordless drill and anything you can find to help secure it in place and spin it by hand.

I used:
- A piece of 2" x 4" wood.
- Some yarn.
- One mixing beater.
- One salad fork.
- A piece of aluminum foil.
- Some scotch tape.

One More Thing You'll Need

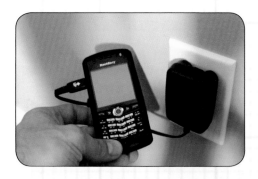

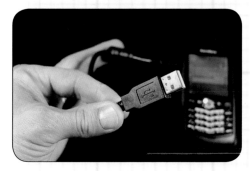

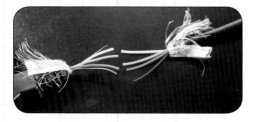

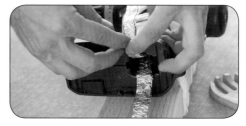

You'll need a way to connect the power you generate to your phone.

Look for an old phone charger you might have and cut it in half. We just need the piece that plugs into the phone. You could even use a USB charger cable like the one I found.

Inside the cable you should see four wires—white, green, red, and black. The red and black ones are the only ones we'll need for this project.

NOTE:

For this project, I used an old Blackberry Pearl. If you are using a smart phone, the white and green wires may need to be shorted out or connected to a "dummy load" to get a successful result (I haven't tested this method yet, but have had feedback from other viewers suggesting this is the case).

Making a Hand-Crank Generator

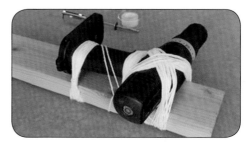

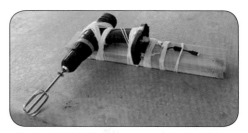

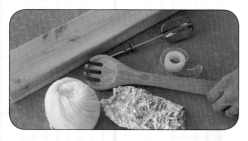

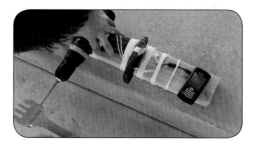

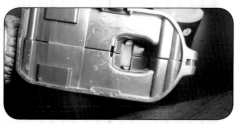

Step 1: Remove the battery from the cordless drill and look up inside. You should see two terminals where the battery provides power to the drill.

Step 2: Use the aluminum foil to fashion makeshift wires that connect to the terminals (salvaged copper wire is even better if you can find some).

Step 3: Secure your drill to a surface like a piece of 2" x 4" with the trigger pressed on. I used plenty of yarn to hold it down tight.

NOTE:

The trigger needs to be on, and the torque setting at its highest.

Step 4: Insert the mixing beater into the drill chuck and make sure it's tightened so the beater won't come out.

Step 5: Add the salad fork through the mixing beater to act as a crank handle and hook up your charger cable. Hook the red wire to the positive lead, and the black wire to the negative lead.

NOTE:

Polarity does matter! If your battery isn't charging, you've probably got the polarity reversed. You can either switch the cables or set your drill to reverse and crank the opposite direction. This will reverse the polarity you generate and should fix the problem.

We've Got Power!

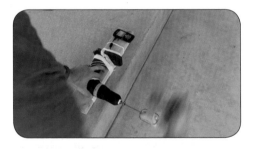

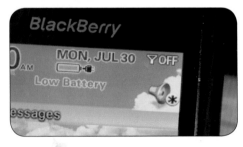

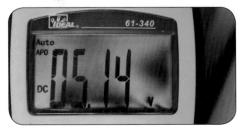

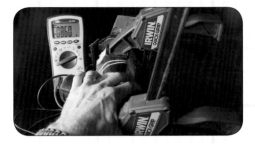

Now all you have to do is twist the rotating end of the drill and you'll be generating electricity at the contact points where the battery would normally connect.

The little plug symbol on this phone appears at around five volts and shows that it's charging. I decided to crank just fast enough to keep the charging symbol displayed to reduce the risk of over-voltage. On my drill, a cranking speed of 100 RPM yielded about five volts DC.

I used some clamps to secure the device to a desk for better leverage. Shorting out the leads on my multimeter returned a value of five to six volts at seven to eight amps. That's a 40-watt human-powered hand-crank generator!

The faster and harder you can crank the drill, the higher the voltage and more amperage you can extract.

Ideally, this could be hooked up to a bike, water power, or even a windmill to generate effortless energy. And if done carefully, the energy could be stored in a battery for later use!

Results

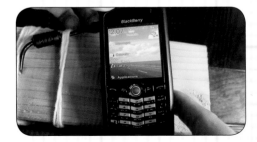

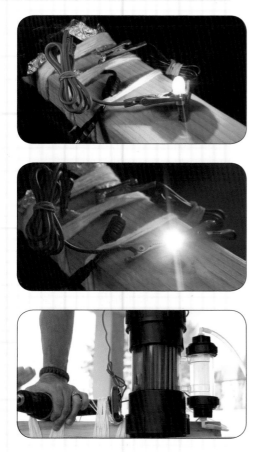

leads are shorted out or hooked up to a rechargeable battery, the effort to crank increases quite a bit! This is because you're pushing more current.

In retrospect, I think it would have been more efficient to spend fifteen minutes cranking a larger current into a large 6-volt battery and then charging the phone from that, but you do what you can with what you have.

The charger illuminated an incandescent flashlight bulb, a super bright white LED, and there was even enough power to convert water into fuel with the OxyHydrogen generator made in a previous project!

Other Projects

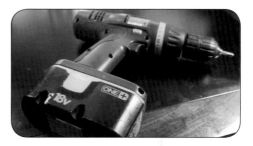

It took about three hours of cranking, but I got my phone fully charged. The phone only accepts a very small current (about 94 mA in my case), so it's not hard at all to crank. But if the generator

Well, there's a bare bones 40-watt electrical generator that you can make in a pinch that will charge batteries, illuminate lights, and provide a little electricity in a pinch.

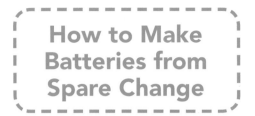

How to Make Batteries from Spare Change

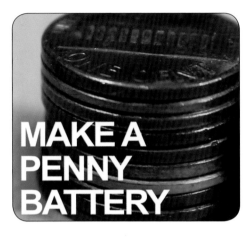

MAKE A PENNY BATTERY

What's a penny worth these days? Not much, but could there be some free energy hidden inside your spare pennies? You'd be surprised! Continue reading to learn how you can put together stacks of pennies to form makeshift batteries that can drive small-current devices like LEDs and calculators.

Step 1: What Kind of Pennies?

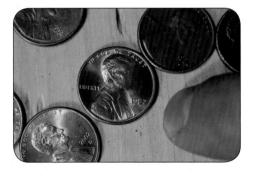

US pennies that are newer than 1982 will work for both of these experiments because they're nearly 98 percent zinc.

Power a Calculator with Three Pennies!

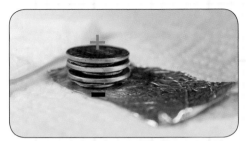

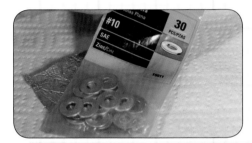

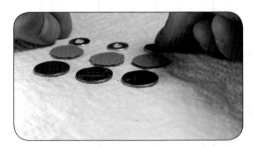

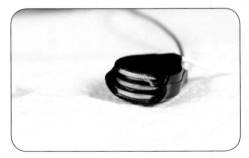

Here's a fun experiment!

Pick up a calculator from the dollar store and remove the screws on the back so you can get to the battery. Remove it and save it for another project.

Now pull the negative and positive leads out of the casing and attach wires to the terminals if you can. I just twisted the wires to the battery leads and used electrical tape to hold them together.

Now it's time to make the penny battery. I found the easiest way to make one is to combine the pennies with some zinc washers from the hardware store. A pack of thirty is about a dollar.

Get some cardboard and cut circular pieces so that the edges are just bigger than the pennies. Let them soak in white vinegar for about one to two minutes.

NOTE:

Any kind of vinegar should work, and if you don't have vinegar, try salt water or lemon juice. They will all work just fine.

Start your battery cell by placing a piece of aluminum foil on your workspace and place one zinc washer at the end. Next, take a piece of cardboard soaked in vinegar, blot dry it on some paper towel, and place it on top of the washer. Lastly, place the copper penny on top of the cardboard, and the battery is done!

An individual battery cell is a zinc bottom, copper top, and separated by a material like paper or cardboard that's been soaked in an electrolyte.

From my testing, each cell yields just over 0.6 volts and around 700mA. The copper top is positive and the zinc bottom is negative. This calculator needs around 1.5 volts, so I used three pennies, three washers, and three pieces of cardboard soaked in white vinegar (three cells x 0.6 volts = approximately 1.8 volts).

I added wires to the top and bottom for ease of use, and then used some electrical tape to hold it together. The aluminum foil is no longer needed.

This type of battery cell is pretty much the same as the first one ever invented by Alessandro Volta in the early 1800s, which came to be known as the "voltaic pile."

Step 3: It Works!

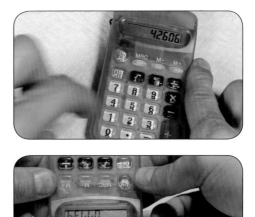

The wires can now be connected to the correct battery leads that were pulled out earlier, and when you press the "on" button, the calculator will fire right up!

I tested out a few functions and everything calculated correctly.

It's amazing to think you can run low-current electrical devices on this penny power hack! It works great, and as long as the cardboard is moist with electrolyte, it should work.

If your battery stops working, try re-soaking the cardboard in a little more vinegar to get it wet, then try again. It should fire right back up!

Making a Larger Wet-Cell Battery

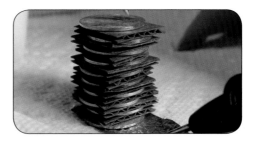

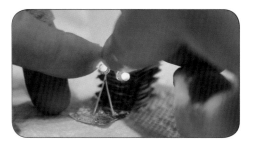

Here's another way to make the battery if you don't have access to zinc washers:

Pick out ten pennies newer than 1982 and use 100-grit sandpaper to sand one face of the penny. The entire inside of the penny is zinc, so sand the face until the whole surface exposes the zinc.

Once again, cardboard needs to be cut and soaked in an electrolyte, like vinegar, salt water, or lemon juice. In this case, I didn't round the edges. You can see the sharp corners, and that's okay as long as they don't touch. If the cardboard pieces touch, that section of the battery will short out and decrease the performance of the unit as a whole.

You can build your battery cells the same way you did with the washers as long as the pennies are all facing the same direction. With this method, the zinc top is the positive and the copper bottom is negative.

By connecting ten cells in series (stacking them on top of each other), the electrical potential will jump to nearly 6 volts! This should be more than enough voltage to drive an LED . . . or TWO!

You can get an LED to light up by pressing the long lead of the LED (positive) on the top and the short lead of the LED (negative) on the aluminum foil base.

LEGALITIES:

Some people have asked about the legality of treating pennies in this manner. The federal law states that there are exceptions made for use as "educational, amusement, novelty, jewelry, and similar purposes as long as the volumes treated and the nature of the treatment make it clear that such treatment is not intended as a means by which to profit solely from the value of the metal content of the coins."

How Long Does an LED Stay On?

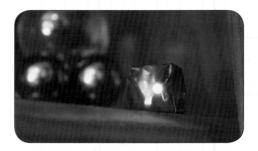

With the stack of ten pennies, I attached a green LED and wrapped it all up with electrical tape in hopes to make it air-tight.

I set it on my shelf and watched it for a few hours to see when it would die out. I was amazed that the light actually stayed lit for over sixteen days! I really am impressed at how well that worked out!

Well, there's an energy idea that's worth a few cents.

Modified Deck of Cards—Looks Normal Enough

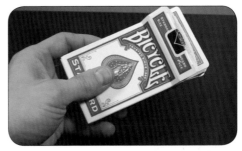

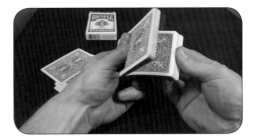

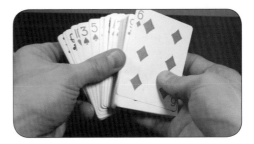

Here's how to make a deck of cards that will pump out a shocking 330 volts of electricity. Stuart Edge used it in his "Electric Shock Kissing Prank" to show the ladies how a man can really put the sparks in a kiss.

WARNING:

This electric shocker outputs around 330 volts DC and delivers a surprising jolt. Be familiar with dangers associated with electric shocks, minor burns, damage to tissues, and possibility of cardiac arrest. This project should not be attempted without adult supervision and adequate training. Misuse or careless use of tools or projects may result in serious injury. Use at your own risk.

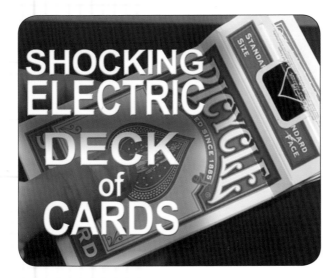

330-volt "shocking" electric deck of cards (electric shock kissing prank)!

This deck of cards may look normal enough, but it has a very shocking secret! 330 volts, to be exact!

I made this gadget for Stuart Edge to use in his "Electric Shock Kissing Prank." Using a magic card trick as a decoy, Stuart and his friend, Kaitlin Snow, got volunteers to kiss them to see if they could "feel the magic." When their lips touched, a 330-volt connection was made and the sparks were flying.

But how does it work? This is how I made it:

stealthy oil tape electrodes are touched by the user and the volunteer, only one more connection needs to be made to complete the circuit. In this case, the circuit is completed with a kiss, and that is where the majority of the electric shock is felt. Have you ever felt magic in a kiss?

Using the deck to charge a capacitor and discharging on a piece of aluminum foil demonstrates the power that can be captured from the device. Here's how to build it:

The Secret Within

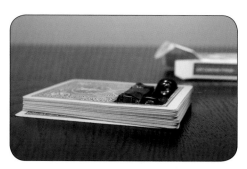

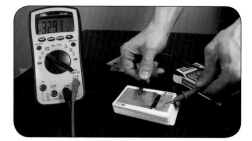

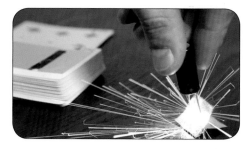

The secret is in the shocker circuit integrated into the deck. When the

The Shocker Circuit

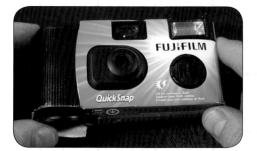

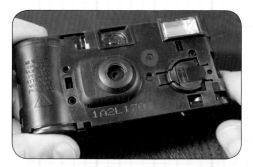

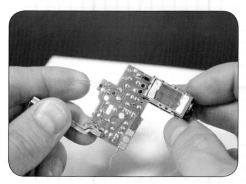

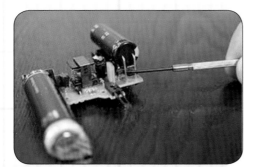

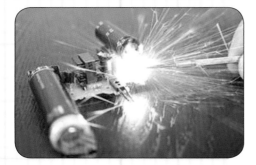

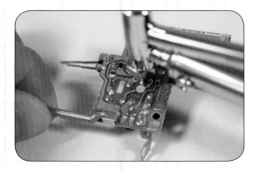

with 330 volts. You'll probably get shocked if you take it out barehanded. To avoid getting shocked, use a piece of metal to short out the two leads on the capacitor, as seen in the pictures.

The circuit needs to be concealed inside the deck, so it has to be made smaller—much smaller. To do this, unsolder the five components and solder the components directly to themselves as depicted. I also chose to add a AAA battery holder and a 1M Ohm tuning potentiometer to adjust the voltage output.

Three wires come off the transformer. One goes to the potentiometer, one goes to battery positive, and the other goes to battery negative and continues on out. This should leave two leads exposed, which will later be attached to the shocker pads.

The last step is to fold some paper around the circuit and fill with copious amounts of hot glue. This should strengthen the components by holding them firmly in place.

Rig the Deck

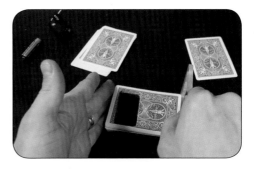

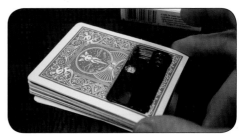

I started by heading to a local drug store and stopping at the photo center. They usually have a whole bin full of disposable cameras ready to be shipped for recycling, and I get them free each time I ask. For this project, I had a FujiFilm Camera, model #1A2L1701. No particular reason for this brand—it's just the one I picked first.

If you want to follow the next steps exactly, you can look for the model number on the outside of the casing.

Opening the case, you'll find a circuit board. This board drives the camera flash and charges an electrolytic capacitor

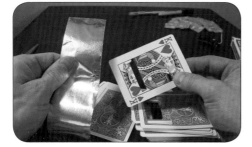

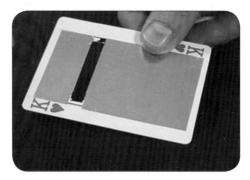

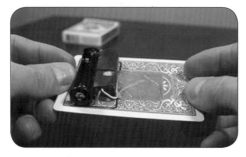

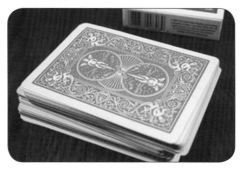

My shocker circuit was the equivalent of forty cards tall, so I used a hobby knife and a plastic template I made to cut all forty cards in a way that would accommodate the circuit. The circuit is a good fit, and because nothing is glued

together, the cards can move freely, giving the illusion that it's just a normal deck.

To make the secret shocker pads, I cut a hole in the bottom card and wrapped conductive foil tape (from most hardware stores) through the hole and around both sides. The shocker circuit sits on top and the wires connect to each respective pad.

NOTE:

The hole needs to be large enough that the pads won't touch each other and short out, and the user needs to be aware that touching them both at the same time will result in an accidental self shock.

The last eleven or twelve cards just sit on top, can shuffle freely, and give the appearance everything is normal. The best part is that it all fits back into the original packaging.

Transfer

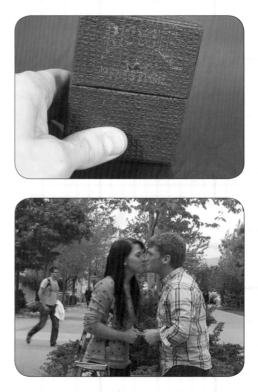

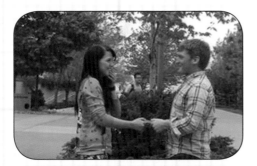

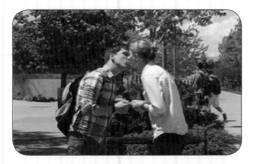

Stuart Edge brought me a nicer carrying case, and it was an easy transfer. Now this gadget was 100 percent ready for his kissing prank video. You can see him holding one side of the cards (one electrode) and the guest holding the other side (opposite electrode). When they kiss, do they feel the magic? You be the judge.

It's important to remember that even though the amount of current flowing in this circuit is extremely low, there may be risks associated with electric shocks. It's important to be aware of the risks and make safety a top concern.

Closing Up

Well, there you have it! That's how to put the electricity in your kiss. Now it's up to you to find your partner.

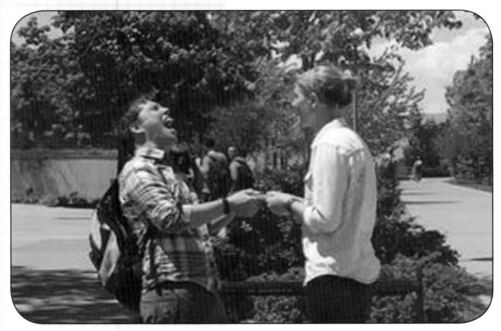

Section 7
Metal Hacks

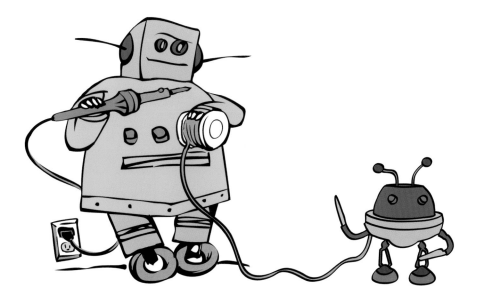

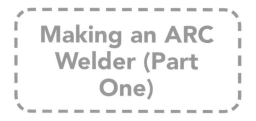

Making an ARC Welder (Part One)

M.O.T. (Microwave Oven Transformer)

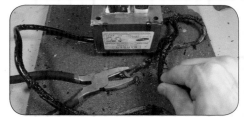

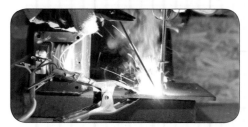

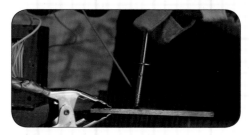

How to convert scavenged microwave parts into a useful arc welding machine. This is part one of two, and focuses on the modification of the transformers.

WARNING:

Stick welding and/or the modification of a Microwave Oven Transformer (MOT) can be very dangerous and presents risks of UV radiation, shock hazards, burns, fires, fumes, and a multitude of other risks. This project should not be attempted without a thorough understanding of electricity, adult supervision, and adequate training. Misuse or careless use of tools or projects may result in serious injury and/or death. Use of this content is at your own risk.

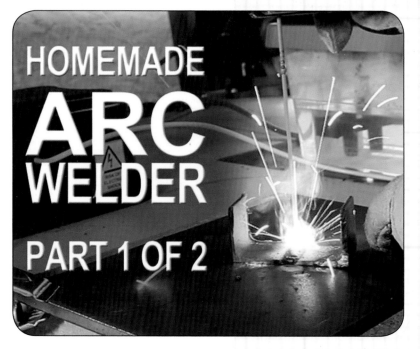

HOMEMADE ARC WELDER PART 1 OF 2

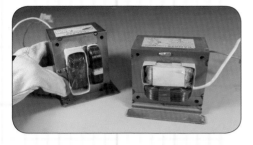

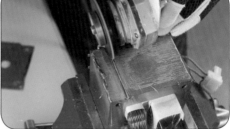

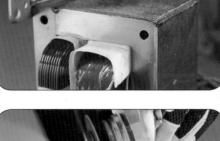

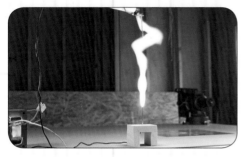

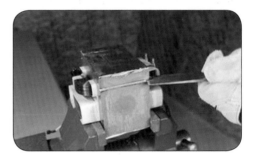

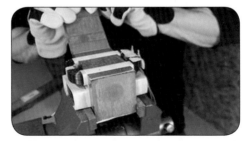

In a previous project, I melted the lead wires on my first metal-melter (page 158). But the transformer core was still in great condition, so I re-used it to make an AC stick welder!

The arc welder made sparks fly, but in the end, it wasn't enough power to make the metal stick, and the welded pieces would break apart with very little effort. If I tried pumping more power into the welder, the wires would overheat and melt.

So, to address this challenge, we'll be using two MOTs (Microwave Oven Transformers) because more transformers mean more power!

Step 1: Transformers Transform

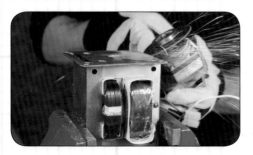

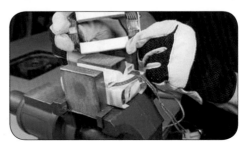

Preparing the MOTs for a new secondary is exactly the same as the first few steps in the Metal Melter project. As it's a little redundant, I won't spend much time on the step-by-step instructions for that, but if you haven't seen it yet, you can reference the Instructable on page 158.

Step 2: A New Secondary

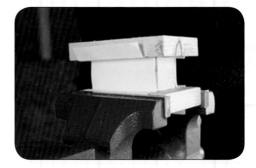

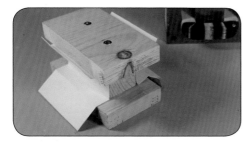

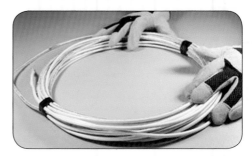

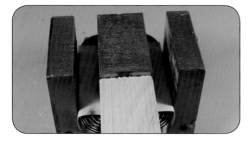

To make life a lot easier, you're going to need to build a little jig for winding your secondary. It's unlikely you'll get all the required turns of wire in such a tight space without one.

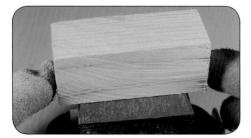

To make this jig, I used a piece of scrap wood and cut it so that it was as wide as the center of the transformer, and just a little shorter than the top. The length was cut so that it overhung about ½" from the ends. I screwed wood panels on the top and bottom to guide the wires and keep them in place, then folded a piece of paper so that it fit in the groove. Once mounted in a bench vice for leverage, the cable can be wound on.

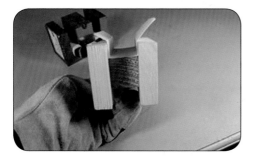

For this project, try to round up around 50' of 8 AWG stranded copper cable from a local hardware store. You could probably save some money by scavenging for free wire, but I decided to look at the "end of coil" section at the hardware store, and was able to negotiate a deal for half price on the cable, so the 50' only cost me about seventeen dollars.

These modified MOTs will need a new secondary that is eighteen turns of the 8 AWG cable, and both M.O.T.s will be tied together in series. I also found I needed to run the system on 240 volts AC to get the power output for good welding. My goal was 30+ volts AC with a variable amperage from 0–120+ Amps.

In practical terms, this means you need to wind the coil on the form so that you end up with six cable lengths high and three cable lengths wide. Oh yeah, and it all needs to be able to fit back in the transformer, so wind it tight!

The first layer isn't too bad, but winding the second layer and third get progressively more difficult and may seem near impossible. Once you get the eighteen turns of wire to fit in the groove, you can fold the paper over, and tape it together to help the coil hold together. Here's the tricky part—get it off the jig without letting it unravel! The top and bottom panels can be removed and the block pushed out from the center of the coil. I used electrical tape to make sure the coils stayed tight.

Step 3: Make the Transplant

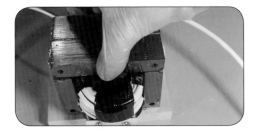

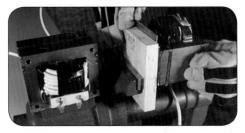

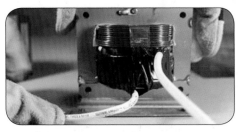

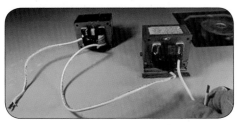

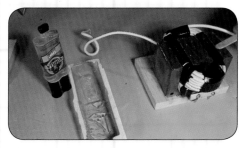

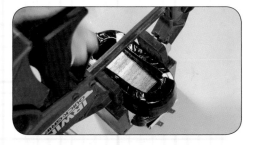

Putting the secondary coil in the transformer is a very tight fit. I had the best success by using a set of clamps to squeeze the sides of the coil in, while I used a rubber hammer to gently tap the coil down.

When it's in, the coil should fit below the top edge of the transformer. Otherwise, you won't be able to get the top back on.

Basically, use two-part epoxy glue to cover the entire top surface, then replace the iron lid and press it together tightly in clamps or a large vice. It's extremely important to have a lot of pressure on the joint while the epoxy is setting. I let mine set for about twenty-four hours.

The modified transformer is complete! The secondary coil is so tight in there that any vibrations from the 60 Hz mains power will be kept to a minimum. When both transformers are modified in the exact same way, we've basically got what we need for welding. All that's left is to clean it up a bit and make it more useful and presentable. By the way, these two exposed wires from the secondaries will become our ground clip and stinger.

Step 4: See Part Two

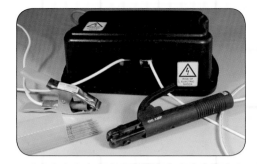

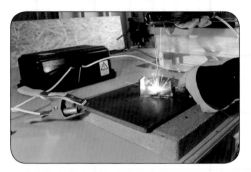

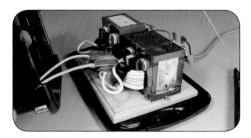

Well, there they are—the basic makings of an AC stick welder!

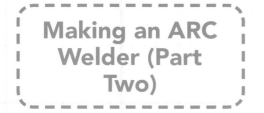
How to convert scavenged microwave parts into a useful arc welding machine. This is part two of two, and it focuses on the electrical system and finishing touches.

WARNING:

Stick welding and/or the modification of a Microwave Oven Transformer (MOT) can be very dangerous and presents risks of UV radiation, shock hazards, burns, fires, fumes, and a multitude of other risks. This project should not be attempted without a thorough understanding of electricity, adult supervision, and adequate training. Misuse or careless use of tools or projects may result in serious injury and/or death. Use of this content is at your own risk.

Step 1: Transformer Platform

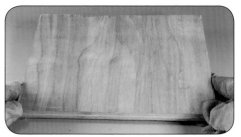

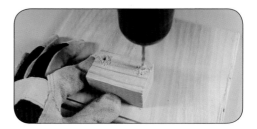

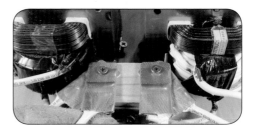

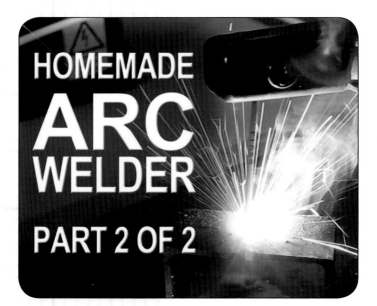

I started this part of the project with a scrap piece of ¾" birch I had left over from my "Router Table" project. The measurements for the board were 7" x 10", and that keeps this about as compact as practical. I found a piece of 2 x 2 as well and screwed it onto the center of the board about an inch from the edge.

Two pilot holes were drilled in the top to accommodate our electrode lugs. I decided to use lugs here rather than keep it all one continuous cable, because it gives the option of changing out electrode cables, or easily modifying the electrical output for future projects.

Step 2: Making and Crimping Copper Lugs

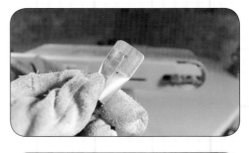

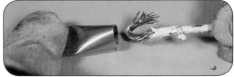

Copper lugs can be pricy, but I found that if I used a 2" length of ½" copper tubing, I could make my own. I used a bench vise to crimp 1" of the tubing completely flat, and then drilled a hole in the flat piece. A belt sander helped to clean up the edges a bit to make it easier to handle, and make it look a bit nicer as well.

For the electrode cables, I used some of the 8 AWG cable left over from when we wound the transformer coils.

Next, I exposed the copper on the end of the cable, and bent it over so it would fit inside the lower part of the lug. I flattened it with a bench vise to make a solid electrical connection, and in my testing, the connection doesn't come apart. If you don't have a bench vise, I imagine a hammer could work with very similar results.

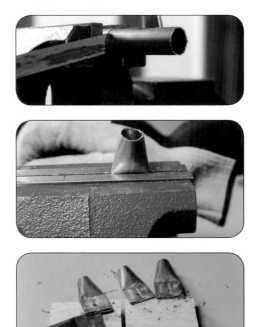

Step 3: Connecting the Electrodes

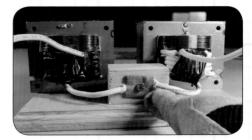

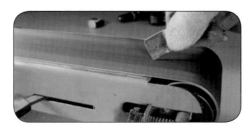

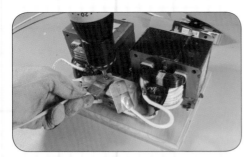

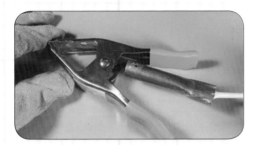

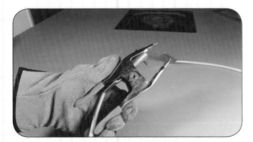

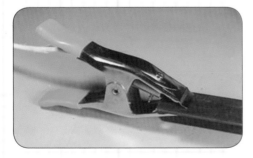

to a common lug so I could have the option to center tap the transformers for future projects, like powering an arc furnace for example.

For the clamp, I found this metal one at the hardware store for only ninety-nine cents. When the rubber tips were removed, it could conduct electricity. I crimped a piece of copper tubing to the wire, and then secured the tube to the clamp with a screw. For being so cheap, the clamp had a surprising amount of clamping force, which was great for biting onto the work piece.

I bought a replacement electrode holder for thirteen dollars rather than making my own. It looked better and was much more practical for welding with.

Step 4: Wiring the Electrical System

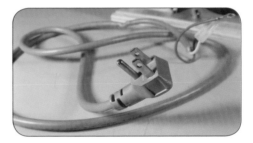

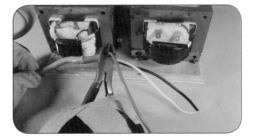

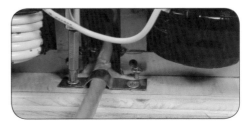

Since the system is AC, there really is no "ground" connection and it doesn't really matter which cable connects to which side, but I decided to put a "ground" clamp on the left side, and the electrode holder on the right.

I also spliced the cable between the two transformers and connected them

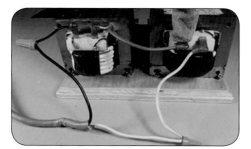

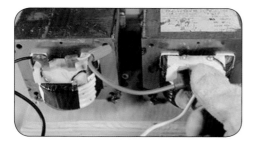

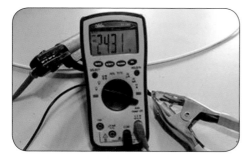

switching the connections on one of the transformers.

I went ahead and did that and ended up with about 37 volts between my ground clip and electrode holder.

Step 5: 240 VAC

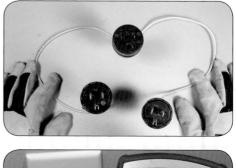

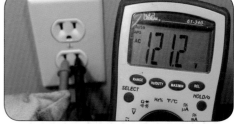

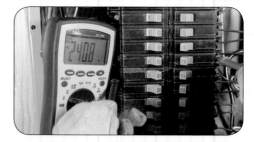

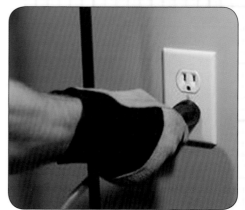

I used one of the cords saved from one of the microwaves and cut off the green wire. I secured the cable to the wood base to prevent the cables from pulling off the connections.

The black cable connects to one of the primary terminals on one of the transformers, and the white wire connects to one of the other transformers primaries. It doesn't really matter which one. I used another piece of wire to connect the other two posts together, essentially connecting the two transformers in series.

Later on, when the device is tested, the two electrodes should be outputting around 36 volts. If you're seeing very low voltage, like 2.4 in my case, that means the transformers are canceling each other out, and this can be fixed by just

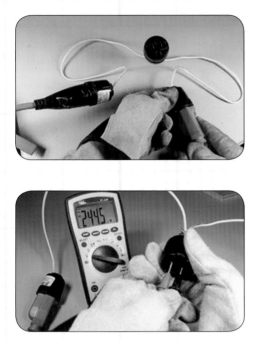

Step 6: Setting the Current

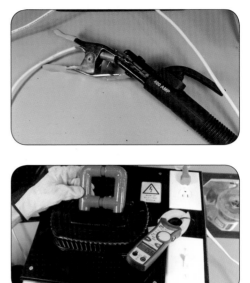

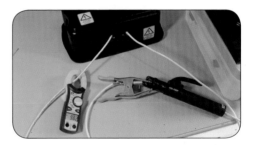

I needed 240 volts AC to power this system, so I used two plugs, a connector, and some 10 AWG wire.

Each of the outlets in my house output around 120 VAC, and the circuits all connect back to the breaker bus bars. There are 2 busses, and I learned that if I took a hot line from each bus, the electrical potential between them was 240 VAC.

Rather than tapping into the breaker box directly, I used extension cords and connected to two different outlets that were 180 out of phase (on separate bus bars). When they were connected to my adaptor, the result was 240 VAC.

It's important to keep in mind that this welder doesn't have an on/off switch and no current limiting of its own. That's why I had to build a separate power controller I call the "Scariac." It's like a "Variac," except much more dangerous. But it is pretty cheap and gets the job done. Look for how to build the Scariac in a different project.

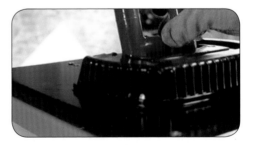

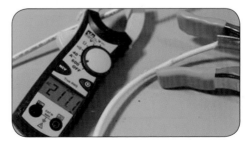

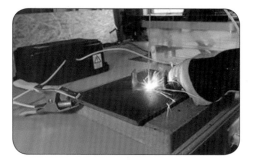

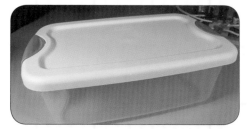

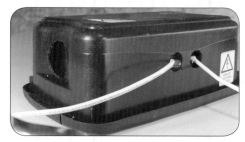

To set the current for welding $\frac{1}{16}$th rods, I connected the ground clamp and electrode holder together, effectively shorting out the system. The Scariac has a loop of wire built in that allows me to monitor the primary current, and when it's set to about 15.5 amps on the primary, it gives me around 100 amps on the secondary.

Cranking up the power on the Scariac can get the welding cables up over 200 amps, but I really don't recommend running them that high for more than a few seconds or the plastic coating on the cables will overheat and may start melting. In any case, you can see there is certainly enough power for welding.

I burned ten $\frac{1}{16}$ rods in a row, and the system was only warm to the touch. This gives me the impression it's got a pretty good duty cycle for use with the smaller rods, and these are probably the only ones I'll really need for my hobby use anyway.

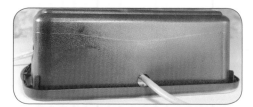

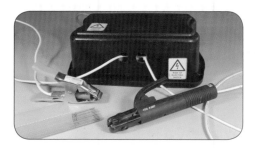

Step 7: Finishing Touches

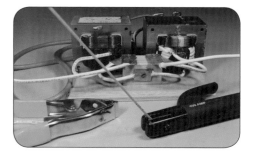

Rather than leaving all the terminals exposed, I picked up a plastic container, painted it black, and drilled a few holes for the cables. I used the top as the base and the bottom as the top. It seemed to work pretty well.

There are also ventilation holes cut in the sides to allow airflow over the coils, and even consideration made for attaching a fan to blow cool air and help regulate the temperature while welding. At this point, the system is completely finished and ready for welding!

Homemade Stick Welder from Microwave Parts!

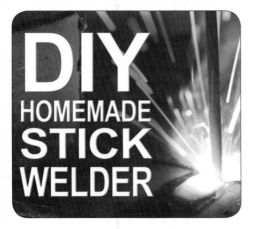

Did you know you can make an AC arc welder using parts from your microwave? I just finished mine, so join me as we put its welding capabilities to the test!

WARNING:

I run the system on 240 VAC, which is metered by a power controller I built called the "Scariac." It's similar to the idea of a Variac (variable auto-controller), but with a few more hazards to be aware of. The Micro-Welder itself does not have an on-off switch, and can pose a fire hazard if plugged directly into a main's power socket. I made this to be used exclusively with the Scariac (look for how to build that in another project). Stick welding and/or the modification of a Microwave Oven Transformer (MOT) can be very dangerous and presents risk of UV radiation, shock hazards, burns, fires, fumes and a multitude of other risks. This project should not be attempted without adult supervision and adequate training. Misuse or careless use of tools or projects may result in serious injury. Use this content at your own risk.

What Is a MOT. Stick Welder?

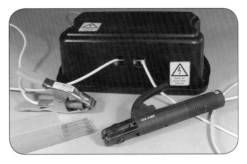

Quite simply, a MOT stick welder is an AC arc welder made by converting/modifying two Microwave Oven Transformers (MOT) so they will weld metal using a welding rod (stick).

A MOT (Microwave Oven Transformer) was modified in a previous project into a spot welder, which is a different form of welder, but in this project I wanted to convert it to arc weld. That requires a different modification, which allows an output of about 30 volts AC and around 120 amps.

I'm happy to say that the welder in this project does work for me. It welds $1/16"$ AC rods very well, and I believe it's very reasonable and sustainable for the amount of welding I plan to do as a simple hobbyist welder.

Disclaimer:

I am not a welder. This project is my introduction into the world of welding, so if you are experienced in welding and metal working, I'm open to suggestions and critiques. However I do ask that you refrain from being overly critical of my welds. They are some of my first. The project is mainly to demonstrate what a welder made from microwave oven parts can do.

Step 2: Quick Project History

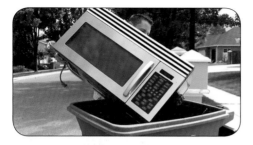

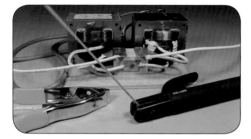

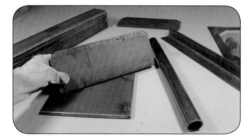

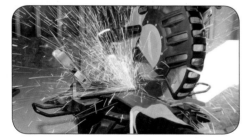

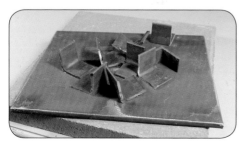

This project started by finding a couple of microwave ovens for free, like I did. Two MOTs were modified so that the output was around 30 VAC and the amperage ranged from 0–120 amps.

I picked up some scrap metal from a welding company down the road and changed out the blade on my miter saw with a 12" metal cutting wheel.

I cut one of the metal pieces into smaller bits so I'd have more pieces I could use to practice welding with.

The MOT stick welder isn't a new idea, but in my experience of trying to duplicate other MOT stick welder projects on the internet, the welder either got so hot that the insulation on the wires melted and shorted it out and/or it didn't provide enough power to strike and maintain an arc. I'm under the impression that up until now, they haven't worked for any practical use.

To date, I haven't seen a video or project where anyone actually welded anything useful with one of these so-called microwave welders. The most that's been shown is to lay a bead on a piece of metal. But this doesn't prove it can weld. My earlier attempts could also lay a bead, but they didn't have enough heat or penetration to make anything stick.

A welder also needs a way to reliably control the amperage (which I haven't seen other projects do). I saw one project where dimmer switches were used on the primary coils. However, dimmer switches are only able to handle around 600 watts, and these stick welders require upwards of 2,000–3,000 watts. In my experience, the dimmer switches fail very quickly.

I don't claim to be the first to make a MOT welder work. My claim is only that this is a way I've figured out that actually does work with satisfying results.

First Welds

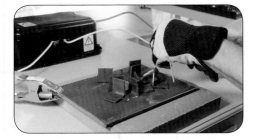

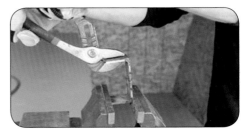

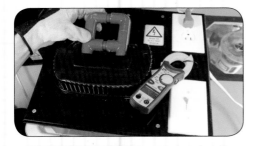

I used one of the large pieces of metal as a base-plate and connected the grounding clip to that.

Using a (6013) 1/16" cellulose-coated rod compatible with AC, I tried making my first welds on two of the pieces I cut earlier.

Striking the arc was like striking a match, and I was happy to see the arc was sustainable. That meant that the voltage and amperage were good.

I regulated the current with a device I call the "Scariac." It works as a current controller to vary the amperage to the welder. Instructions can be found on page 118.

When the slag was knocked off the weld, the only way I really had of testing it was a destructive test—bending it until it broke.

I placed the metal in my bench vice and bent it all the way over. I was actually surprised when the weld held strong. Success!

I tried the same thing with another piece, and did eventually get the metal to rip, but it tore below the weld. The welds never did break!

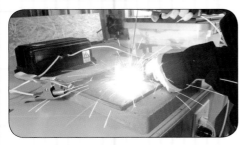

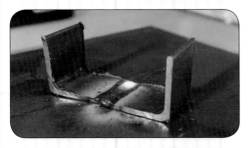

Second Opinion

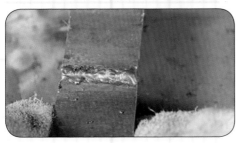

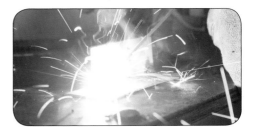

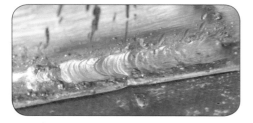

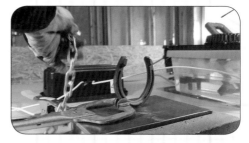

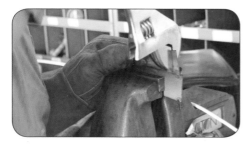

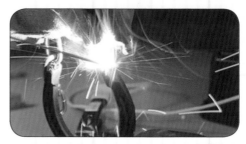

I took my unit to a friend who actually is an experienced welder. I wanted to get a more professional opinion. He tested it out on some stainless steel, and gave some great feedback.

His experience was that the weld completely penetrated the metal, and he said it worked as well as the one he had in his shop. We tried breaking the weld, and again proved it held fast. The metal outside the weld tore, but the bead didn't.

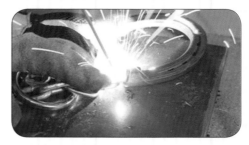

More Welding for Practice

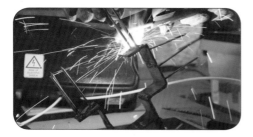

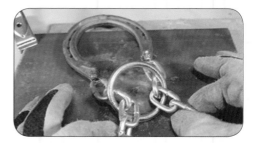

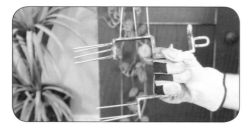

For extra practice, I welded all the small pieces of metal and anything else I had lying around. Some framing nails and chain got included, and pretty soon I had some metal art that looked something like a weapon for a zombie apocalypse.

I also tried making the classic horseshoe puzzle using two horseshoes, some lengths of chain, and a 2" steel ring. It worked out pretty well!

The goal is to try and get the ring off, which seems impossible because it's too small, but I let my wife play around with it and she proved it can be done.

Additional Features

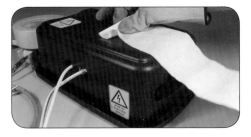

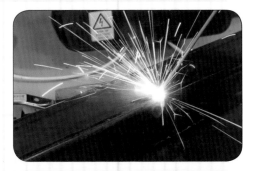

I tried welding with some larger $\frac{3}{32}$" rod, but the welder started to overheat fast. The welds required much more current, which made the coils get hot and put them in danger of melting.

I probably wouldn't use this to weld with $\frac{3}{32}$" on a regular basis, but to combat the extra heat, I used a fan salvaged from one of the microwaves and placed it up to a vent hole in the side of the welder's casing. This blows air over the coils and exhausts the air out the other side. In the event of extreme overheating, the entire top can be removed for maximum cooling.

Success!

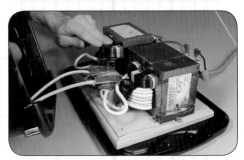

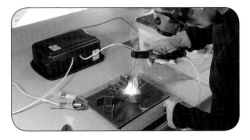

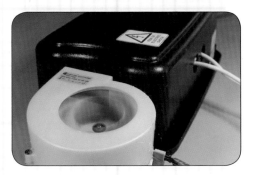

Well, there it is! A MOT stick welder that is proven to work!

How to Make a Spot Welder for Cheap!

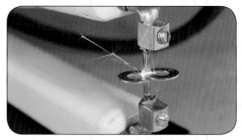

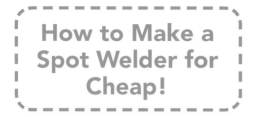

A typical resistance Spot-Welder can range in price from about $200 to $800, but with a little resourcefulness and a bit of free time, you can make one like this for about $10 or less.

Spot welders are used to fuse thin sheets of metal together. They are most likely used in the auto industry as well as HVAC for welding metal ducting.

You Might Be Surprised How Cheap It Can Be

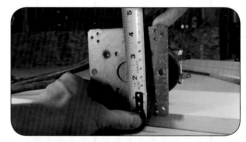

Step 1: Take Some Measurements

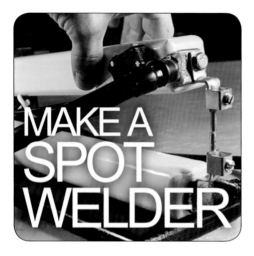

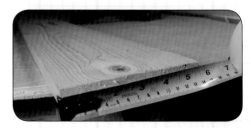

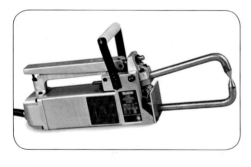

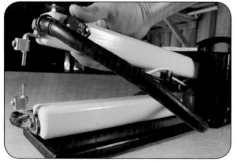

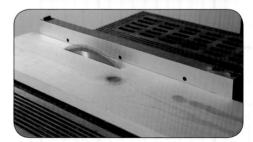

Measuring the base of my Metal Melter, I found it was about 4¼".

I found a six-foot length of 1x6 common board for about four dollars, which actually measures out at 5½", so it will work just fine.

Two pieces of the board will need to be cut to 12" lengths (5½" x 12"), but the rest can be pushed through a table saw to trim the width down to 4½" (¼" wider than the transformer base).

Step 2: Roughing the Case Together

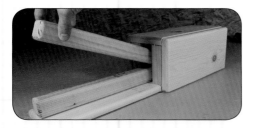

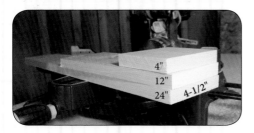

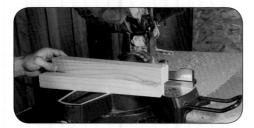

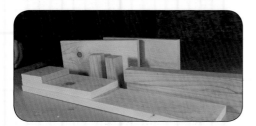

The piece of common board that you just trimmed down to 4½" wide can be cut into three pieces measuring:

- 4" x 4½"
- 12" x 4½"
- 24" x 4½"

The other two pieces of the common board should measure:

- 12" x 5½" (x two pieces)
- You'll also need four pieces of 2x2 measuring:
- 2" x 2" x 13½" (x two pieces)
- 2" x 2" x 4" (x two pieces)

This is all the wood you'll need for building the casing.

I used a ¾" rounding bit and my router to smooth the edges and give it a cleaner look.

This is roughly how it will look when it's assembled.

Step 3: Prepping the Pieces

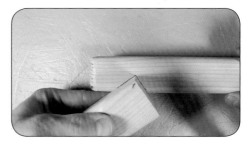

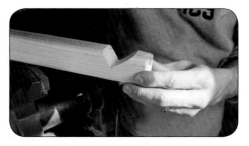

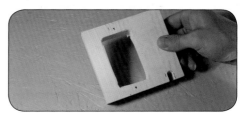

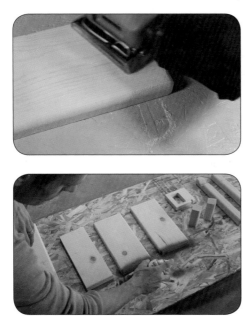

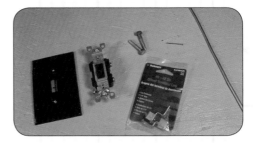

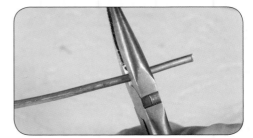

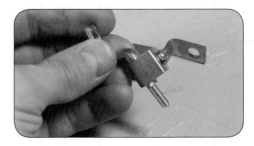

A notch needs to be cut on one of the 2x2 arms, and you'll see what this is for later on. I found that a piece of scrap can be used as a template.

The notch can be cut out with a band saw, wood saw, or any other saw you can get creative with. I used a jigsaw, but wouldn't recommend it as the safest option.

The back panel (4" x 4½") also gets holes cut that will accommodate an electrical light switch and a notch for a power cable.

The pieces get sanded, primed, and painted. I chose to paint this black and yellow.

Step 4: Additional Materials

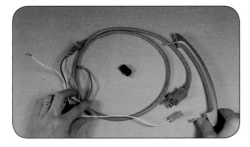

When I salvaged the Microwave Oven Transformer in a previous project, I saved some of the other components that can be used for our Spot Welder:

- The power cord.
- The door handle.
- Wires for the transformer terminals with insulated spade connectors.
- Power switch with wires and insulated spade connectors.

Aside from these, the only other items you'll need are:

- Simple light switch, with faceplate
- Copper offset terminal lugs that will hold (x two).
- ¼" hex screws (x two).
- Small nails (x two).
- Length of solid copper wire (4 AWG is better, but I used 6 AWG in this project).

The solid copper wire can be snipped into 1" lengths that fit nicely into the terminal lugs.

The lugs have a mechanism that can be tightened with a screwdriver to secure the connection with the wire. The tighter, the better.

Step 5: Start Assembly

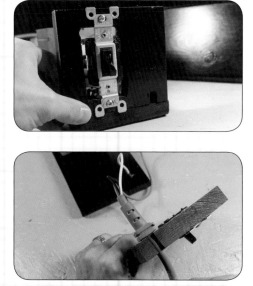

Now that the wood is painted, finished, and dry (I gave it about two days), the unit can be assembled.

The back panel is for a light switch and a power cord.

Before screwing the panel into the base, make sure your cord goes in first. The thick piece at the end of the cord prevents it from pulling back though the hole.

This is also the time to add the two pieces of 2" x 2" x 4" support blocks to the base. Be sure of your measurements before you screw them down. You want them to end up flush with the side panels when it's done.

The Metal Melter can be placed inside now, and when a good position is found, it can be screwed to the base with a couple of small screws.

Now it's time to wire up the electrical system.

Step 6: The Electrical System

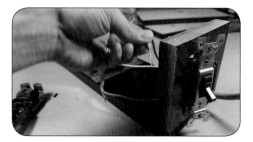

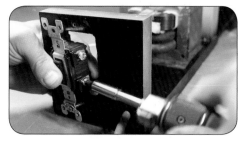

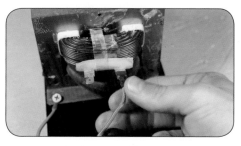

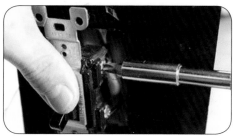

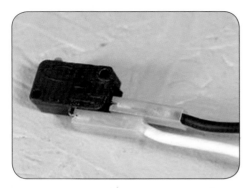

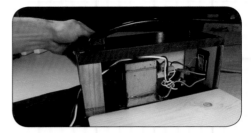

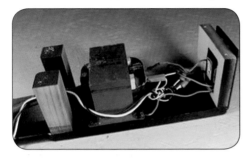

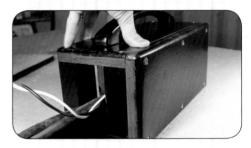

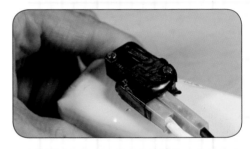

Starting with the power cord coming into the casing, I stripped the black wire and attached it to the bottom terminal of the light switch.

Next, I attached one of the wires I had salvaged to the right terminal on the transformer, stripped the other end, and attached that to the top of the light switch.

The electrical could almost be finished here, but I wanted to add another switch for safety and convenience, and that's where the salvaged switch from the microwave hack comes in.

The two wires attached to the switch can be wrapped with electrical tape to secure the connection and help insulate from electric shock.

Then both ends of the wires are stripped so the copper wire is exposed.

One wire connects to the left terminal of the Metal Melter's primary coil, and the other wire connects to the white wire on the power cable that runs back to the house.

The electrical system is complete!

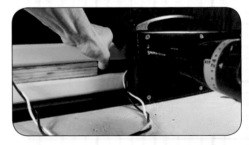

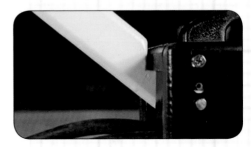

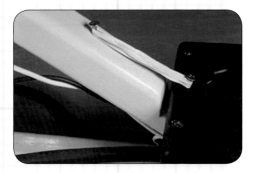

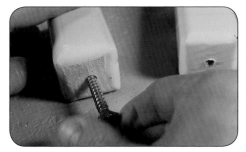

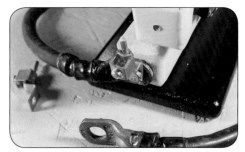

The sides can be screwed on with six wood screws on each side. I used 2" wood screws after drilling pilot holes to make sure the wood didn't split.

The trigger switch is attached near the tip of the top welder arm and at a bit of an angle, so it can be pressed easily. I found that two small nails held this in place perfectly.

Both arms can get inserted into the front of the casing, and with a bit of guesswork, a hole can be drilled through the side of the casing and into the end of the arms so that when a nail is inserted, it will pivot.

Now you can see why we needed the notch in the arm.

To help the arm stay in an upright position, I added a couple of screws and rubber bands to keep the tension.

This also provides a little back pressure and stabilization when using the welder.

Step 8: Adding the Electrodes

The copper lugs can be added to the tips of the arms.

I drilled pilot holes with a $\frac{3}{16}$th drill bit, then secured the lugs by pushing the hex bolts first through the hole in the lugs, then through the lugs on the Metal Melter terminals—one in the top and one in the bottom. It shouldn't matter which way they go, but I chose to make my top cable on the same side as the switch because it was easier to handle.

If the electrode tips don't line up perfectly, it's easy to bend them a little until they do.

Step 9: The Finished Result

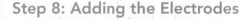

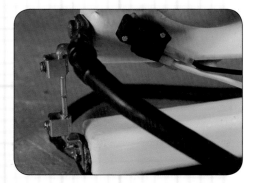

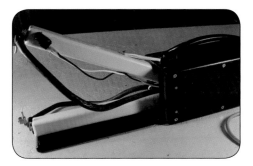

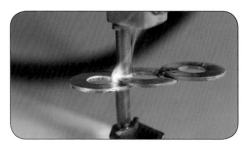

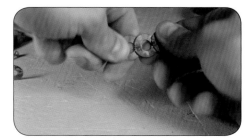

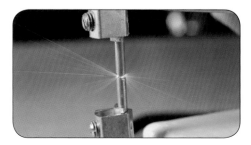

When the energized electrode tips touch each-other, you can see the high-amp sparks.

NOTE:

Burning galvanized metals may release zinc-oxide fumes. Welding should be done in a well ventilated area.

Step 10: Additional Features

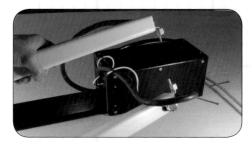

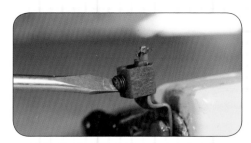

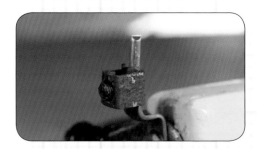

The Spot Welder is finished!

It will only work if the safety switch on the back is turned on, and even then, no power is delivered until the thumb-operated switch is pressed.

To use, place thin sheets of metal between the electrode tips, then press the button with your thumb for about three or four seconds.

The massive electrical current pushing through the metal heats it up to the point where it fuses with the other sheet.

You can release your thumb from the switch and wait until the weld cools enough to handle.

Welding these metal washers worked so well that I couldn't break them by hand. I had to use two pairs of pliers to get them to snap.

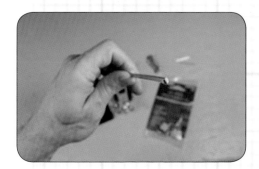

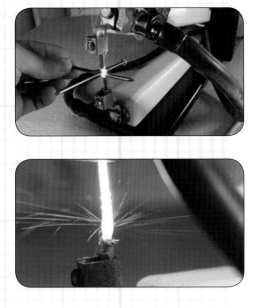

The electrode arms are only held in with nails, so if the nails are removed, the arms can be removed to extend the welders reach and access difficult angles.

They go back together very easily and the elastic can be conveniently replaced when necessary.

When the electrode tips are spent, it's easy to unscrew the bolt holding them in place and add a fresh piece of copper wire.

Copper wire is relatively cheap. You can get a piece of 12" 4 AWG wire for about a dollar. That means each tip is less than ten cents each!

The power of the metal melter is still evident in the way this can bring iron metal to a boil! Be careful running the welder too long, because there is a chance the wires will get so hot that the insulation on the cables will start smoking and melt.

Now you know how to make my version of a cheap Spot Welder.

How to Make the Metal Melter

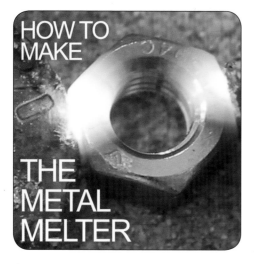

In this project you'll learn step by step how to modify a microwave oven transformer into a high-current device that can pump out 800 amps of electrical current.

If you liked the Metal Melter you saw in a previous project, here's how you can make your own!

Step 1: Find an Old Microwave

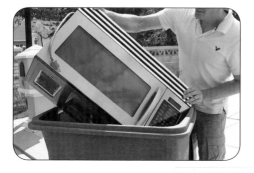

Start by finding an old microwave for free—the bigger, the better.

You can find them in various places, like on free classified ads or in your neighbor's garbage can, like where I found this one.

Step 2: Harvest the Transformer

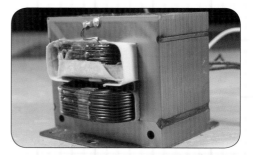

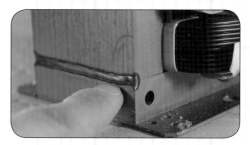

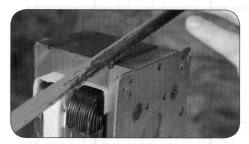

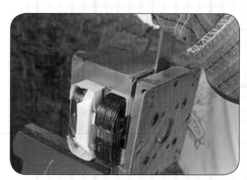

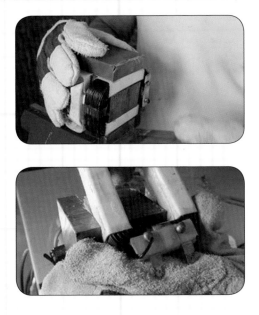

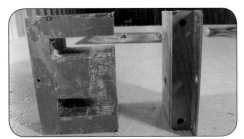

Step 3: Rewind the Coils

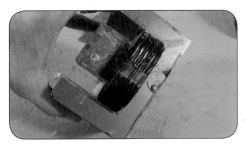

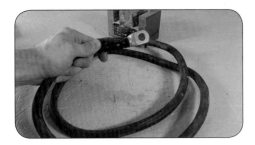

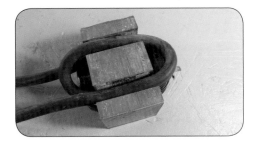

The transformer is the piece that you'll need, and it looks like this.

CAUTION:

Make sure you're familiar with the dangers of opening a microwave because there are components inside that may still carry a charge and could hurt or even kill you—even if the microwave isn't plugged in.

The transformer core is only held together by two very thin welds, as seen on the side of this one.

A hacksaw or angle grinder can be used to cut the weld, and then a hammer and chisel can be used to break it open, giving you access to the primary and secondary coils.

Be very careful taking the primary coil out, because you'll need it again. Make sure not to bend, break, or scratch it in any way.

NOTE:

The secondary coil is harder to get out, and may be damaged by the time you do, but that's ok because we don't need it for this project. However, if you can salvage it intact, it may be a source of thin gauge enameled copper wire for future projects.

Okay, your transformer core should now be bare. These are the "E" and "I" sections of the core, and have been scraped with a chisel to remove glue and paper stuck to the insides.

The next step is to carefully replace the primary coil and ensure it's snug at the bottom of the core. After that, add

159

a 5' length of 2 AWG insulated copper cable. This thicker cable will extend the amount of time a massive electrical current can flow before the cable overheats.

The secondary cable is only wrapped one and ¾ times around the center.

Step 4: Glue It Back Together

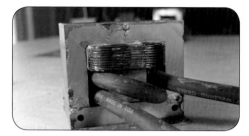

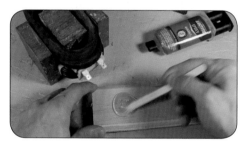

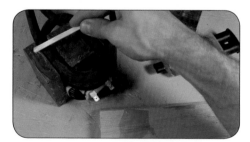

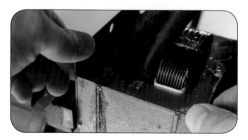

If you don't have a way to weld the base back on, you can use some two-part

epoxy-glue and apply to all the surfaces that will be in contact.

After that, clamp it together to let the glue set. I used my bench vise as a clamp and it worked perfectly!

When the glue is dry, none of the wires should be touching each other, but what it can do is very impressive.

Step 5: Melt Some Metal

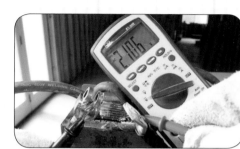

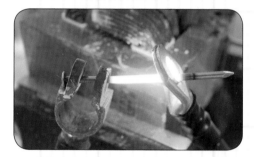

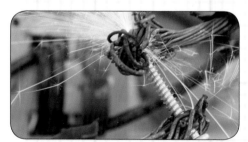

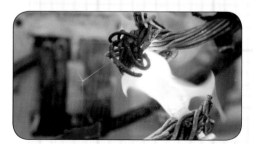

The output voltage on this is just barely over two volts, but the amps are closer to 800! That's enough current to melt iron nails and steel bolts on contact!

Step 6: Spot Welder

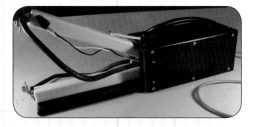

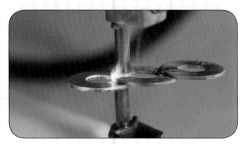

I found a practical use for The Metal Melter in making a Spot Welder like this one. The electrical current can be concentrated to a single point to fuse thin sheets of metal together. This is known as a "spot weld."

You can see how I made this in a different project.

Now You Know!

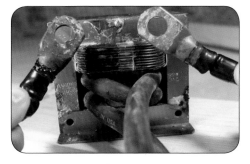

Now you know how to make the Metal Melter!

Section 8
Miscellaneous Hacks

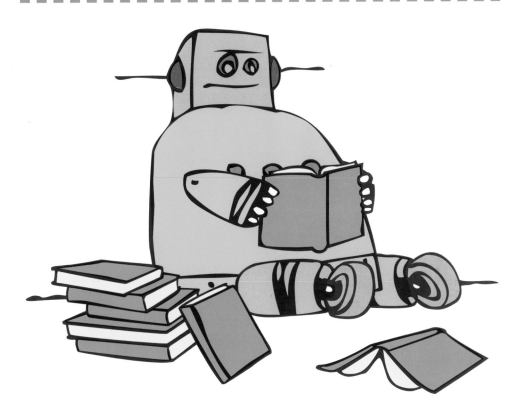

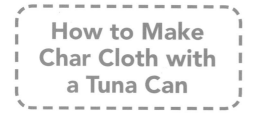

How to Make Char Cloth with a Tuna Can

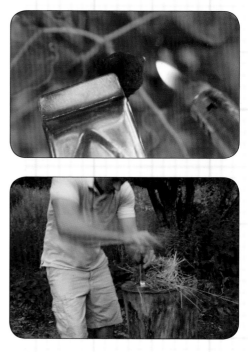

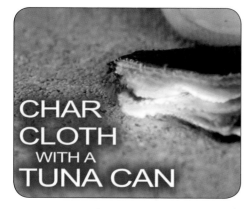

I sacrificed my kids' clothes and a can of tuna to make some high-quality fire starter! Here's how to make a great batch of char cloth to add to your emergency kit.

WARNING:

This project should not be attempted without adult supervision and adequate training. Misuse or careless use of fire and flammable materials may result in serious injury, property damage, and/or death. Use of this content is at your own risk.

What Is Char Cloth?

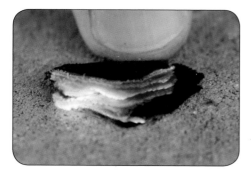

Char cloth is fire-starting tinder that has the ability to capture and hold a spark amazingly well, and for a considerable amount of time.

According to Wikipedia:

"Char cloth (also called charpaper) is a swatch of fabric made from vegetable fiber (such as linen, cotton or jute) that has been converted via pyrolysis into a slow-burning fuel of very low ignition temperature.

It is capable of being ignited by a single spark that can in turn be used to ignite a tinder bundle to start a fire.

It is sometimes manufactured at home for use as the initial tinder when cooking or camping and historically usually provided the 'tinder' component of a tinderbox. It is often made by putting cloth into an almost airtight tin with a small hole in it, and cooking it in campfire coals until the smoking slows and the cloth is properly charred.

Char cloth ignites with even the smallest spark, and is therefore commonly used with a flint and steel."

Step 1: Materials You'll Need

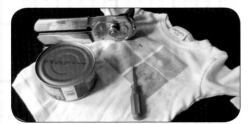

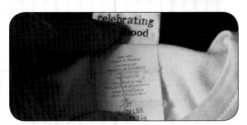

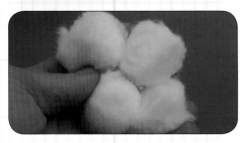

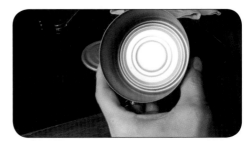

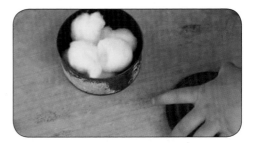

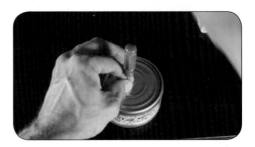

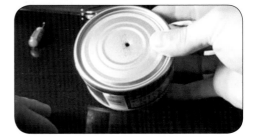

This project can be done with items you probably already have around the house!

- Tuna Can
- "Lid lifter" style can-opener
- Nail, punch, or small screwdriver
- Cotton fabric

For cotton fabric, old T-shirts work very well if they're 100 percent cotton. You can find this information on the tag inside the shirt. I also found that cotton balls work extremely well, and have become my new favorite!

Step 2: Cook the Cotton

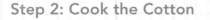

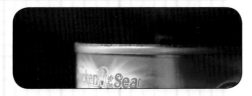

To make the char cloth cooker, just follow these steps:

1. If possible, use a "lid-lifter" style can-opener to open the can. This cuts the top off along the side of the can.
2. Clean out your tuna can and make sure it's dry and free of contaminants.
3. Place four to eight cotton balls inside the can (or about four round pieces of cotton fabric from your T-shirt).

4. Replace the lid and press it back into place (note: If you cut it with a "lid-lifter" style can opener, it should press and hold together like it was meant to be!).
5. Flip the can over and use your punch to make a small hole in the "top" of the cooker.

Your cooker is complete and ready to go!

Step 3: Fire It Up!

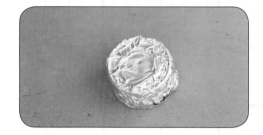

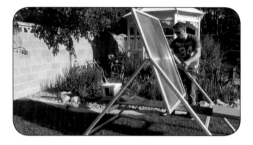

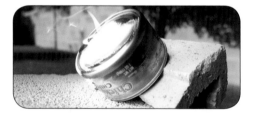

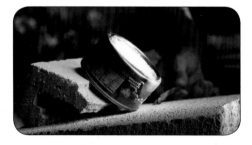

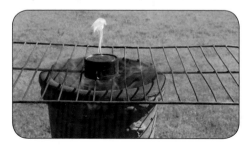

The goal is to heat the container up over 752°F (400°C), which can be done in a variety of ways. For example:

- Use solar power
- Place directly in an open flame.
- Any other outdoor method of inducing heat (outdoors because potentially harmful gases will be released and can smell up your house).

When the container gets hot enough, the cotton releases gases, including hydrogen and methane gases. As these gases are cooked out, the fiber becomes carbonized through a process called "pyrolysis." This means that the fiber is charred but not burned.

You can tell the process is working because you'll see the gas venting through the hole in the top of the container. These gases are flammable and may ignite. Don't worry if they do because that's normal and just fine.

The cooking is done when the gas stops and the flame goes out.

NOTE:
I've found that cooking them beyond the point where the gases stop and flame goes out can negatively affect their performance, so take the container off the fire as soon as possible.

Next:

- Place a layer of aluminum foil over the hole to prevent air from sucking back into the container.
- Let cool for about five minutes.

NOTE:
The container is very hot, so use protection on your hands to avoid being burned while applying the foil.

How Did It Turn Out?

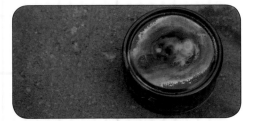

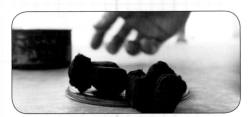

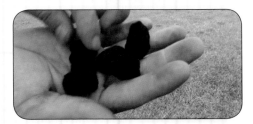

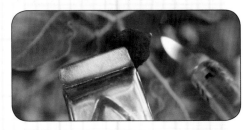

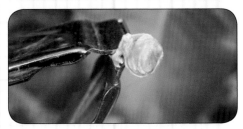

When the container has cooled off completely, open it up and the first thing you'll hopefully see is that your white cotton fabric or cotton balls have turned completely black.

NOTE:

If there are parts that are still white or brown, it's not cooked completely and needs more time on the fire.

To test your batch of char cloth, brush gently with an open flame. The cloth should capture the heat and form a small spark that will continue to smolder for an impressive amount of time. One cotton ball can last a couple of minutes.

By blowing air onto the spark, heat will transfer quickly and can engulf the entire cloth. This is the great advantage of the cloth. It can deliver a lot of heat when you need it (by blowing on it) or just hold a spark for a couple of minutes while you're getting your tinder bundle ready.

In Closing

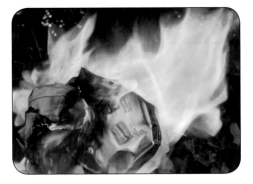

Well, there's how to make a batch of char cloth using materials from around the house. It's great for emergencies, so go make a batch for your emergency kit right now!

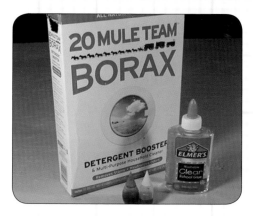

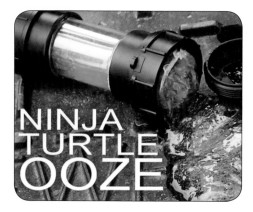

Hey, look at this! There's a broken canister of mutant ooze leaking down into the sewers! But don't worry because this sticky slime is non-toxic, and it's so easy to make, a three-year-old can do it!

Step 1: Gather These Materials

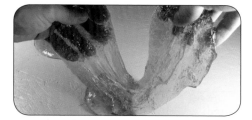

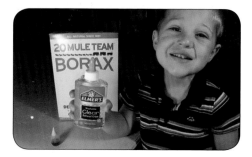

Inspired by Dr. Anne Helmenstine with About.com, my kids and I found and slightly modified a recipe for making slime.

My kids went crazy for it! It's great stuff because it's basically harmless and extremely easy to make. So easy, in fact, that my little three-year-old did it himself (with a little coaching, of course).

If you'd like to make it at home, here's how we did it!

Step 2: Gather Your Materials

You will need:

- ½ teaspoon borax laundry booster (found in grocery stores in the laundry detergent section).
- 5 ounces clear school glue (usually in the craft section of some grocery stores, or stores like Walmart).
- Green and yellow food coloring.
- Water.

Step 3: Make the Solutions

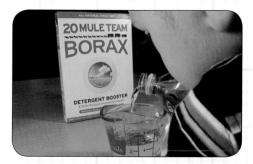

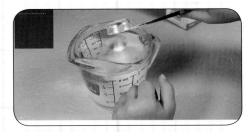

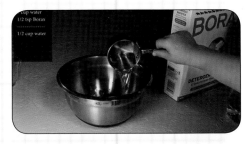

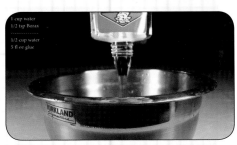

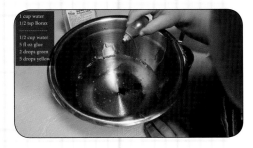

Step 4: Mix the Solutions

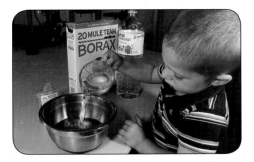

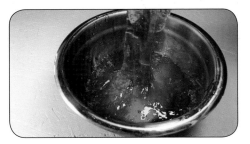

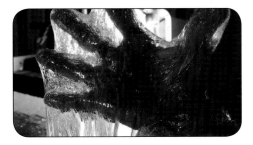

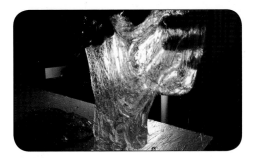

Make Solution "A"

In one container, mix:

- 1 cup of warm water
- ½ tsp of borax

  Stir to dissolve as much as possible.

Make Solution "B"

In a separate container, mix together:

- ½ cup of water
- Entire 5 ounce bottle of clear glue
- Stir in 2 drops of green food coloring
- Stir in 5 drops of yellow food coloring

Pour solution "A" into solution "B." And right before your eyes will magically appear a gooey green flubber!

Holding this in front of a light makes it look like some sort of creepy alien experiment!

Step 5: Make a Cool Ooze Canister

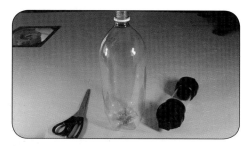

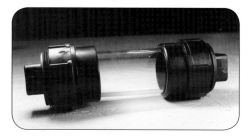

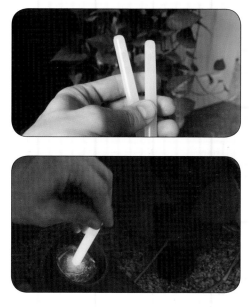

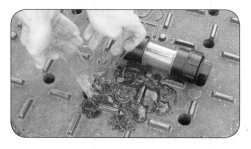

I wanted to make a fun container for this ooze, and using these materials, I came up with this one.

Materials:
- 2 black 2" ABS clean-out adaptors.
- 2 black 2" ABS plugs from Home Depot.
- For the tube:
- 2" tube of acrylic (7" tall) works best. OR
- Plastic soda bottle.

Step 6: Make It Glow

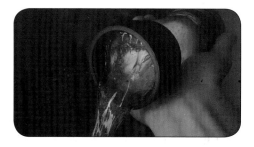

With the ooze inside the container, I tried adding a yellow glow stick to see what effect it would have.

It made the slime glow an eerie green light and makes it look radio-active!

I also noticed that putting the glow stick in the microwave for four seconds could make it glow three times as bright!

Step 7: Other Projects

That's how to make your very own Ninja Turtle Ooze.

How to Make a Gravity Puzzle (Brain Game)

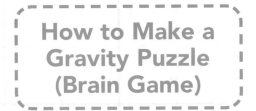

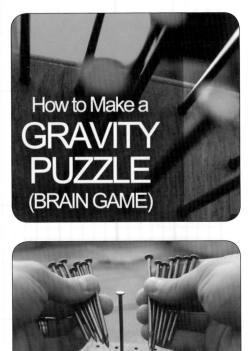

Step 1: A Look at the Finished Project

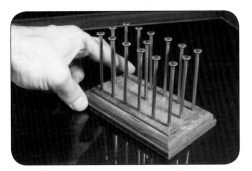

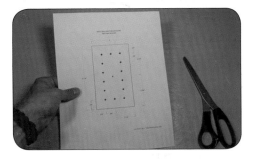

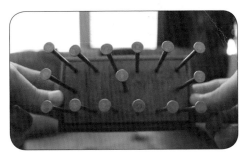

This little brain game is all about engineering a lower center of gravity. The idea has been around forever, but most people still can't do it. The challenge is simple; just balance these fourteen nails on one nail head. The nails can't touch anything except each other, and they all have to be balancing at the same time.

In this project, you'll learn how to make a fun little mind puzzle for giving as a gift or for entertaining guests. You'll also learn the secret to getting all these nails to balance at once!

All this project really needs is about fifteen framing nails (3" work well) and something to hammer one of them into. It's as easy as that!

However, to make this into a proper project, you're going to need to glorify the idea a little by making a nice presentation stand.

I used a simple spreadsheet program to make a template that would accommodate the fifteen nails on a board of wood with one nail right in the center.

Step 2: Make the Nail Base

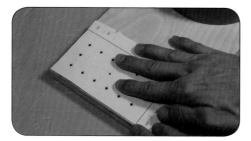

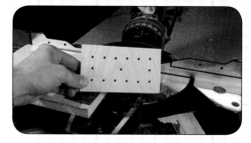

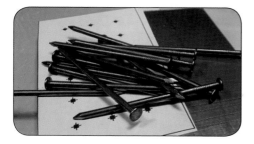

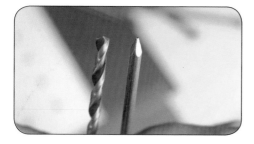

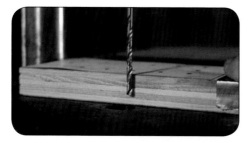

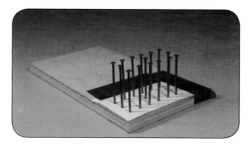

I found a piece of scrap wood at a local hardware store (Home Depot) that they just gave me for free, but they will usually sell scrap pieces for about fifty cents each.

By taping the template to the top of the wood, it's quick and easy to make the cuts and drill the holes. There are fifteen holes in the template to accommodate fifteen framing nails. It's important that the nails have flat heads at the top. You'll see why later on.

We want holes that allow us to manipulate the nails in and out, but small enough to prevent them from flopping around. I found that a $\frac{9}{64}$" drill bit worked perfectly with these nails.

When drilling the holes, make sure you don't drill all the way through the wood unless you plan to glue another piece to the base. I used a drill press to gauge the depth of the holes, and after drilling all the holes, I inserted nails to make sure all the tops were level.

Now the edges can be cut. I used a chop saw to make the cuts, and at this point you are finished with the template. The paper can be removed and thrown away.

To make the nail base look more professional, I used my router table and a beading bit to sculpt the edges, then some fine sandpaper to clean it up and get it ready for staining.

I used a rosewood stain because it's what I had on hand. Two coats of stain went on, letting it sit for three minutes before wiping off the excess, and then finishing it with some shellac to add some gloss and seal the wood.

At this point, you should have a nail base that looks like the one in the pictures.

It might seem like a lot of work, but it's really pretty simple. And remember, you can use this as a decoration piece or a game for entertaining guests, so take some pride in your work!

After it's dried for a couple of hours, it's finished and ready to use on your friends!

Step 3: Alternative Nail Bases (If you're feeling lazy)

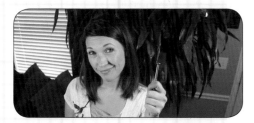

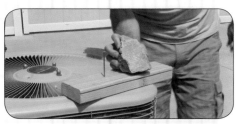

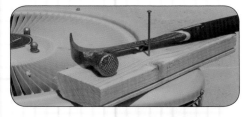

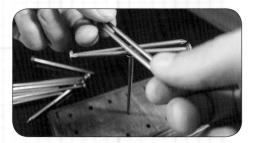

Of course if you're feeling lazy or don't have the tools to put this much work into the project, you can just use a hammer and a scrap piece of wood.

If you don't have a hammer, maybe you can find a rock? If you don't have wood, hammer, or a rock, hopefully you have someone who likes you enough to just hold the nail upright? It's really that easy.

Now for the challenge!

Balance the remaining fourteen nails on this one nail head. The nails can't touch anything except each other, and they all have to be balancing at the same time.

While this trick has probably been around since before any of us were born, most people still don't know how to do it!

Step 4: Solving the Puzzle

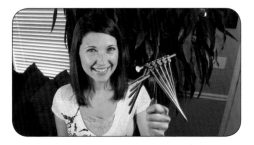

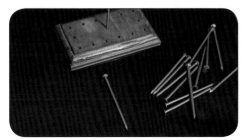

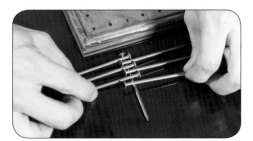

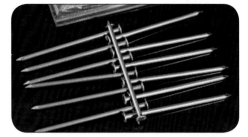

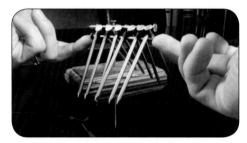

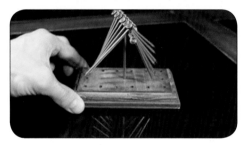

other nails drape down, binding their heads on the top overlaying nail.

From here, it's easy to balance the entire contraption on the lone nail head.

The center of gravity is now lower than the balancing point, so this structure is fairly stable and resists falling when it's bumped, blown on, or tapped.

For another challenge, see if you can balance fifteen wooden matches like this. It's much harder, but once they balance, they are amazingly stable as well!

One More Challenge

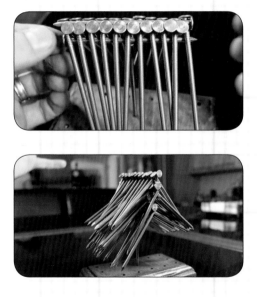

Have you tried to solve the puzzle on your own yet?

You may want to give it a go before seeing the solution. This is one of those puzzles that seems impossible until you learn the super simple pattern that makes it work, then it's easy!

Solving the puzzle:

Start by placing a nail on the table and staggering the other nails on top so they alternate directions, as seen in the pictures, and so that there is just enough room between the opposing heads so that the last nail can be laid down on top. This last nail faces the opposite direction to the first one laid on the table.

Now you can take the nail on the bottom and slowly lift upwards until the

I found that when the contraption is balancing, the nails could be pushed closer together and more nails could be added. I got each unit up to twenty-three nails!

The next question was how many could be stacked on top of that?

I repeated variations of this pattern and stacked four units of about twenty-two nails each for a total of eighty-nine nails balancing at once!

How many can you get?

Turn a Mousetrap into a Powerful Handgun

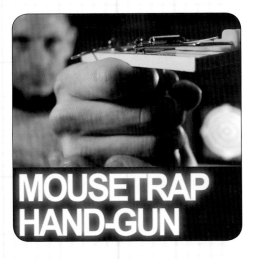

Here's how to turn a mousetrap into a fun little handgun that shoots up to forty feet! This is a great project because it can be made with simple materials, with very basic tools, and in just a few minutes!

Step 1: What You Will Need

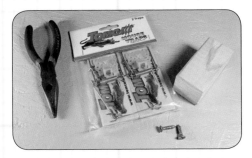

This pack of two mousetraps was only ninety-eight cents from Lowes home improvement store!

Aside from those, all you're going to need are:

- Two small screws (like the kind on your door hinges)
- A small piece of 2x2
    Suggested tools to make the job easier are:
- Screwdriver
- Needle-nose pliers
- Wire snips

Step 2: Prepare the Mousetrap

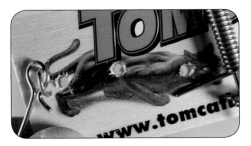

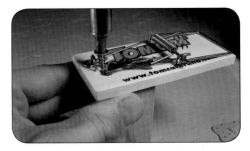

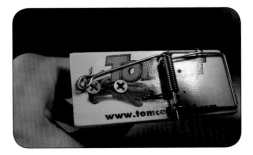

Cut the piece of wood so that it fits comfortably in your hand, and then drill three holes with a ⅛" drill bit in the places shown in the picture.

The two screws will secure the trap to the wood handle. Make sure you leave just a little overhang at the back.

Step 3: Make the Firing Mechanism

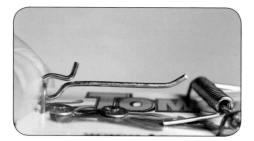

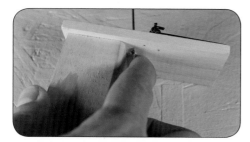

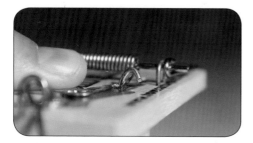

The firing mechanism is made by modifying the locking pin into a squeeze-pull trigger.

Modify the locking pin so that it's trimmed down in a way that it overlaps the most forward hole you drilled, and then bend the tip of the pin up at a 45-degree angle.

The next step is to use the locking pin from the other trap as the trigger. Push the pin up through the bottom of the hole, then trim it flush with the top of the spring and bend it over in an "n"

shape. This will prevent it from slipping back down through the hole.

Step 4: Add the Launching Pad

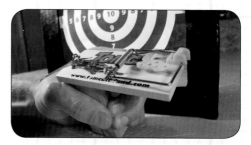

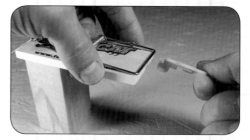

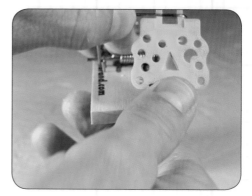

The bait pad can be converted into a launching platform that will shoot any type of small ammunition!

With the trap hammer relaxed, clip the bait pad with the hooks facing upward, and then carefully lift the hammer, tuck the pad underneath, and relax the hammer back down onto the trap base.

Your gun is finished and ready for testing!

Step 5: Loading the Mousetrap Gun

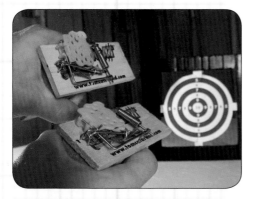

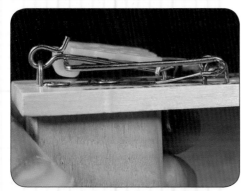

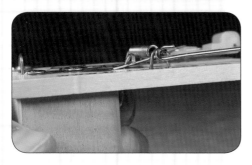

To cock the gun, pull the hammer back in the same way you would set the mousetrap. Carefully overlap the locking pin and set the tip so that it holds firm in the hook you made on the trigger pin.

Be careful with this step and make sure your fingers are clear, because if the pin slips, the trap hammer will snap over and give your fingers a smack.

I made a little target for practice. In the next step, you'll see different types of ammo that work well for shooting.

Step 6: Types of Ammunition

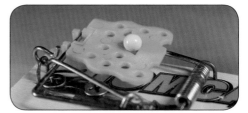

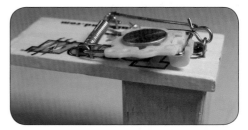

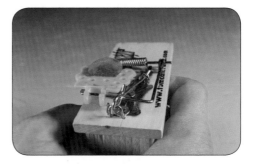

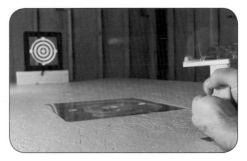

I found that Airsoft BBs work perfectly! The little divot in the center of the pad is perfectly situated to shoot these BBs straight forward and at distances up to forty feet! They are small, fast, and don't do too much damage to anything they hit.

Other types of ammunition I found work well are:

- Pennies
- Small rocks
- Plastic bottle caps
- Glass beads

Basically, any item that's small and dense works great!

Moving the ammo forward on the pad makes the gun shoot low and fast, like a gun. Shifting the ammo rearward causes the object to be launched high and far, like a catapult.

You can play around with different positions to see how your shooting patterns are affected.

Step 7: Finished

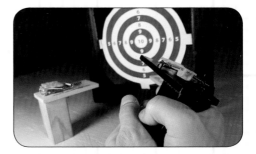

This simple device launches projectiles with both power and precision. Cost was about a dollar.

Just for fun, I made a third gun and painted it black to see how it would contrast with the yellow launch pad.

CONVERSION TABLES

One person's inch is another person's centimeter. Instructables projects come from all over the world, so here's a handy reference guide that will help keep your project on track.

Measurement								
	1 Millimeter	1 Centimeter	1 Meter	1 Inch	1 Foot	1 Yard	1 Mile	1 Kilometer
Millimeter	1	10	1,000	25.4	304.8	—	—	—
Centimeter	0.1	1	100	2.54	30.48	91.44	—	—
Meter	0.001	0.01	1	0.025	0.305	0.91	—	1,000
Inch	0.04	0.39	39.37	1	12	36	—	—
Foot	0.003	0.03	3.28	0.083	1	3	—	—
Yard	—	0.0109	1.09	0.28	033	1	—	—
Mile	—	—	—	—	—	—	1	0.62
Kilometer	—	—	1,000	—	—	—	1.609	1

Volume									
	1 Milliliter	1 Liter	1 Cubic Meter	1 Teaspoon	1 Tablespoon	1 Fluid Ounce	1 Cup	1 Pint	1 Quart	1 Gallon
Milliliter	1	1,000	—	4.9	14.8	29.6	—	—	—	—
Liter	0.001	1	1,000	0.005	0.015	0.03	0.24	0.47	0.95	3.79
Cubic Meter	—	0.001	1	—	—	—	—	—	—	0.004
Teaspoon	0.2	202.9	—	1	3	6	48	—	—	—
Tablespoon	0.068	67.6	—	0.33	1	2	16	32	—	—
Fluid Ounce	0.034	33.8	—	0.167	0.5	1	8	16	32	—
Cup	0.004	4.23	—	0.02	0.0625	0.125	1	2	4	16
Pint	0.002	2.11	—	0.01	0.03	0.06	05	1	2	8
Quart	0.001	1.06	—	0.005	0.016	0.03	0.25	.05	1	4
Gallon	—	0.26	264.17	0.001	0.004	0.008	0.0625	0.125	0.25	1

conversion tables

Mass and Weight						
	1 Gram	1 Kilogram	1 Metric Ton	1 Ounce	1 Pound	1 Short Ton
Gram	1	1,000	—	28.35	—	—
Kilogram	0.001	1	1,000	0.028	0.454	—
Metric Ton	—	0.001	1	—	—	0.907
Ounce	0.035	35.27	—	1	16	—
Pound	0.002	2.2	—	0.0625	1	2,000
Short Ton	—	0.001	1.1	—	—	1

Speed		
	1 Mile per hour	1 Kilometer per hour
Miles per hour	1	0.62
Kilometers per hour	1.61	1

Temperature		
	Fahrenheit (°F)	Celsius (°C)
Fahrenheit	—	(°C x 1.8) + 32
Celsius	(°F − 32) / 1.8	—

also available

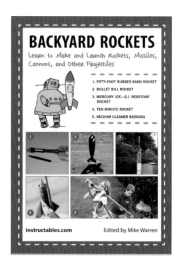

Backyard Rockets
Learn to Make and Launch Rockets, Missiles, Cannons, and Other Projectiles

by Instructables.com, edited by Mike Warren

Originating from Instructables, a popular project-based community made up of all sorts of characters with wacky hobbies and a desire to pass on their wisdom to others, *Backyard Rockets* is made up of projects from a medley of authors who have collected and shared a treasure trove of rocket-launching plans and the knowledge to make their projects soar!

Backyard Rockets gives step-by-step instructions, with pictures to guide the way, on how to launch your very own project into the sky. All of these authors have labored over their endeavors to pass their knowledge on and make it easier for others to attempt.

US $12.95 paperback ISBN: 978-1-62087-730-2

also available

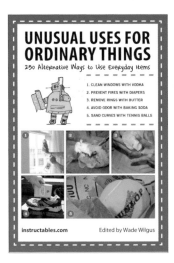

Unusual Uses for Ordinary Things
250 Alternative Ways to Use Everyday Items
by Instructables.com, edited by Wade Wilgus

Most people use nail polish remover to remove nail polish. They use coffee grounds to make coffee and hair dryers to dry their hair. The majority of people may also think that the use of eggs, lemons, mustard, butter, and mayonnaise should be restricted to making delicious food in the kitchen. The Instructables.com community would disagree with this logic—they have discovered hundreds of inventive and surprising ways to use these and other common household materials to improve day-to-day life.

Did you know that tennis balls can protect your floors, fluff your laundry, and keep you from backing too far into (and thus destroying) your garage? How much do you know about aspirin? Sure, it may alleviate pain, but it can also be used to remove sweat stains, treat bug bites and stings, and prolong the life of your sputtering car battery. These are just a few of the quirky ideas that appear in *Unusual Uses for Ordinary Things*.

US $12.95 paperback ISBN: 978-1-62087-725-8

also available

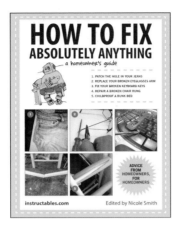

How to Fix Absolutely Anything
A Homeowner's Guide
by Instructables.com, edited by Nicole Smith

There are a million things that can go wrong in your home. Faucets leak. Floorboards creak. Paint flakes. Chairs break. With *How to Fix Absolutely Anything*, you'll have step-by-step instructions to tackle even the most confounding repairs in your home, including:

- Installing a toilet
- Replacing the belts on your washer and dryer
- Patching up a hole in the wall
- Bringing a power adapter back to life
- Re-covering chairs
- Getting wax out of your carpet
- And many more!

From changing lightbulbs to fixing a kitchen cabinet hinge, *How to Fix Absolutely Anything* is a collection of the most indispensable advice and tips from people across the world who face the same problems you do. Hundreds of color photographs and easy-to-follow instructions make this book perfect for all levels of experience. It's a no-brainer for any homeowner, and the one gift to get any friend, family member, or loved one living on their own for the first time. Broke the microwave handle and don't know what to do? With *How to Fix Absolutely Anything*, the solution is only a few pages away.

$16.95 paperback ISBN: 978-1-62914-186-2

also available

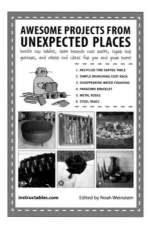

Awesome Projects from Unexpected Places
Bottle Cap Tables, Tree Branch Coat Racks, Cigar Box Guitars, and Other Cool Ideas for You and Your Home
by Instructables.com, edited by Noah Weinstein

Awesome Projects from Unexpected Places features more than thirty projects designed by the users of instructables.com. These users have repurposed and reused everyday items they've found around their homes, in their backyards, or even in local junkyards to create unique furnishings and decorations for their homes and meaningful gifts for others. These projects are at the core of the maker movement and can inspire us all.

Readers will learn how to construct:

- Bottle cap tables
- Concrete lamps
- 3D string art
- Sand fire gardens
- Screw-nut and wooden rings
- Paracord bracelets
- Cigar box guitars
- Wooden beer mugs
- Test tube spice racks
- Metal roses
- And more!

US $12.95 paperback ISBN: 978-1-62087-705-0